Supporting the Mental Health of Migrant Children, Youth, and Families

Editors

MARGARET CARY
JOSHUA D. FEDER
ALISON MONDS WARD

CHILD AND ADOLESCENT PSYCHIATRIC CLINICS OF NORTH AMERICA

www.childpsych.theclinics.com

Consulting Editor
JUSTINE LARSON

April 2024 • Volume 33 • Number 2

ELSEVIER

1600 John F. Kennedy Boulevard • Suite 1800 • Philadelphia, Pennsylvania, 19103-2899

http://www.theclinics.com

CHILD AND ADOLESCENT PSYCHIATRIC CLINICS OF NORTH AMERICA Volume 33, Number 2
April 2024 ISSN 1056–4993, ISBN-13: 978-0-443-13031-1

Editor: Megan Ashdown
Developmental Editor: Shivank Joshi

Child and Adolescent Psychiatric Clinics of North America (ISSN 1056-4993) is published quarterly by Elsevier Inc., 360 Park Avenue South, New York, NY 10010-1710. Months of issue are January, April, July, and October. Business and Editorial Offices: 1600 John F. Kennedy Boulevard, Suite 1800, Philadelphia, PA 19103-2899. Periodicals postage paid at New York, NY and additional mailing offices. Subscription prices are $373.00 per year (US individuals), $100.00 per year (US & Canadian students), $424.00 per year (Canadian individuals), $487.00 per year (international individuals), and $200.00 per year (international students). For institutional access pricing please contact Customer Service via the contact information below. International air speed delivery is included in all *Clinics* subscription prices. All prices are subject to change without notice. **POSTMASTER:** Send address changes to *Child and Adolescent Psychiatric Clinics of North America*, Elsevier Health Sciences Division, Subscription Customer Service, 3251 Riverport Lane, Maryland Heights, MO 63043. **Customer Service: 1-800-654-2452 (U.S. and Canada); 314-447-8871 (outside U.S. and Canada). Fax:** 314-447-8029. **E-mail:** JournalsCustomerService-usa@elsevier.com **(for print support) or** journalsonlinesupport-usa@elsevier.com **(for online support).**

Reprints. For copies of 100 or more of articles in this publication, please contact the Commercial Reprints Department, Elsevier Inc., 360 Park Avenue South, New York, New York 10010-1710 Tel.: 212-633-3874; Fax: 212-633-3820, E-mail: reprints@elsevier.com.

Child and Adolescent Psychiatric Clinics of North America is covered in *MEDLINE/PubMed (Index Medicus), ISI, SSCI, Research Alert, Social Search, Current Contents,* and *EMBASE/Excerpta Medica.*

Contributors

CONSULTING EDITOR

JUSTINE LARSON, MD, MPH, DFAACAP
Medical Director, Schools and Residential Treatment, Consulting Editor, *Child and Adolescent Psychiatric Clinics of North America*, Sheppard Pratt, Rockville, Maryland, USA

EDITORS

MARGARET CARY, MD, MPH
Medicaid Behavioral Health Medical Director, Oregon Health Authority, Child and Adolescent Psychiatrist, Yellowhawk Tribal Health Center, Portland, Oregon, USA

JOSHUA D. FEDER, MD
Editor in Chief, *The Carlat Child Psychiatry Report*, Executive Medical Director, Positive Development, Co-Chair, Disaster and Trauma Issues Committee, AACAP, Solana Beach, California, USA

ALISON MONDS WARD, MD
Team Lead–Mental and Behavioral Health Services, Division of Health for Unaccompanied Children, Office of Refugee Resettlement, US Department of Health and Human Services, Washington, DC, USA

AUTHORS

MAWUENA AGBONYITOR, MD, MSc
Office of Refugee Resettlement, Washington, DC, USA

V. KARINA ANAYA, MD
Keck–USC Voluntary Adjunct Clinical Assistant Professor of Psychiatry and the Behavioral Sciences, Co-Director Refugee Health Alliance

ABISHEK BALA, MD, MPH, Central Michigan University, Saginaw, Michigan, USA

BEVERLY J. BRYANT, MD
Co-Chair, American Academy of Child and Adolescent Psychiatry Committee on Child Maltreatment and Violence, Child Psychiatry, Talkiatry, McKinney, Texas, USA

LEEALLIE PEARL CARTER, MD
PGY4 Child and Adolescent Psychiatry Fellow, Mountain Area Health Education Center in Asheville, NC in partnership with the University of North Carolina, Asheville, North Carolina, USA

LINDA CHOKROVERTY, MD, FAAP
Attending Psychiatrist, Psychiatric Observation Suite, Departments of Psychiatry and Behavioral Sciences, and Pediatrics, Montefiore Health Systems, Albert Einstein College of Medicine, Bronx, New York, USA

VANESSA C. D'SOUZA, MD
Department of Psychiatry and Psychology, Mayo Clinic, Rochester, Minnesota, USA

JOSHUA D. FEDER, MD
Editor in Chief, *The Carlat Child Psychiatry Report*, Executive Medical Director, Positive Development, Co-Chair, Disaster and Trauma Issues Committee, AACAP, Solana Beach, California, USA

LISA R. FORTUNA, MD, MPH
University of California Riverside, Psychiatry and Neurosciences, Riverside, California, USA

EMILY HOCHSTETLER, MD
University of Massachusetts, T.H. Chan School of Medicine, Worcester, Massachusetts, USA

RACHEL KRONICK, MD, MSc, FRCPC
Assistant Professor, Division of Social and Transcultural Psychiatry, McGill University, Montreal, Quebec, Canada

KEVEN LEE, PhD
Postdoctoral Fellow, Division of Social and Transcultural Psychiatry, McGill University, Montreal, Quebec, Canada

SARAH L. MARTIN, MD
Texas Tech University Health Sciences Center, El Paso, El Paso, Texas, USA

PETER METZ, MD
Professor of Psychiatry and Pediatrics Emeritus, University of Massachusetts, T.H. Chan School of Medicine, Worcester, Massachusetts, USA

DIANA MICONI, PhD, MA
Assistant Professor, Department of Educational Psychology and Adult Education, Université de Montréal, Outremont, Montréal, Quebec, Canada

ANUSHAY J. MISTRY, MD
Children's Hospital Los Angeles, Los Angeles, California, USA

JESSICA PIERCE, MD, MSc
University of Michigan, Ann Arbor, Michigan, USA

KAREN PIERCE, MD, DFAACAP, DLFAPA
Department of Psychiatry, Northwestern University, Chicago, Illinois, USA

MICHELLE V. PORCHE, EdD
University of California San Francisco, Psychiatry and Behavioral Sciences, San Francisco, California, USA

CÉCILE ROUSSEAU, MD, MSc
Professor, Division of Social and Transcultural Psychiatry, McGill University, Montreal, Quebec, Canada

GEORGINA SANCHEZ-GARCIA, PhD
The University of Texas at El Paso, College of Health Sciences, El Paso, Texas, USA

JEANETTE M. SCHEID, MD, PhD
Associate Professor, Psychiatry, Michigan State University, East Lansing, Michigan, USA

SUZAN SONG, MD, MPH, PhD
Boston Children's Hospital, Boston, Massachusetts, USA

OMAR TAWEH, BS, BA
University of Massachusetts, T.H. Chan School of Medicine, Worcester, Massachusetts, USA

LEECIA WELCH, JD
Deputy Litigation Director, Children's Rights, New York, New York, USA

Contents

Upholding the Human Rights and Well-Being of Refugee Children Through Effective Clinical Care   111

Lisa R. Fortuna and Michelle V. Porche

> Refugee children are often exposed to adversities and traumatic experiences that can harm the mental health and well-being of refugee children. These include human trafficking and exploitation and dangers in detention centers and refugee camps. All these adverse events can be traumatic and contribute to poor mental health, including posttraumatic stress, anxiety, depression, and substance use disorders. Therefore, the assessment of refugee children and adolescents should include screening and identification for these experiences, provision of evidence-based trauma treatment, and social supports to promote their well-being and thriving.

Cultural Considerations and Response to Trauma for Displaced Children at the Border   125

Georgina Sanchez-Garcia, Beverly J. Bryant, and Sarah L. Martin

> The United States has long been the leading destination for Latin Americans seeking refuge. However, in the last 7 years, many children from Mexico and northern Central America, composed of El Salvador, Honduras, and Guatemala, have joined this migratory flow. The experience of forced migration is intense, chronic, and complex for children in their home countries, during their journey, and on arrival in the United States. Their stories can inform clinical practices, such as Psychological First Aid and Trauma-Focused Cognitive Behavioral Therapy, to promote resilience in children in vulnerable conditions.

Unaccompanied Children in the Office of Refugee Resettlement Care   141

Mawuena Agbonyitor

> Unaccompanied children entering the United States are cared for in a variety of care provider settings across the country while they are in the custody of the Office of Refugee Resettlement (ORR). While in an ORR care provider program, children receive physical and mental health-care services, classroom education, social skills/recreation services, vocational training as appropriate, family unification services, access to legal support, and case management. The Mental and Behavioral Health Services Team was created in 2019 to provide oversight of the mental health of unaccompanied children in ORR care.

events they encounter. This includes determining if premigration, migration, and postmigration stressors have had an impact on the individual. This has also helped clinicians, educators, and legal advocates to use a collaborative approach to address the migrant youth's needs for managing the severity of PTSD symptoms.

Migrant youth commonly access mental health care for the first time during emergencies, rather than through ambulatory means. Suicidal behaviors may occur more often among migrants than nonmigrant youth, and they may suffer from post-traumatic stress, depression, anxiety, and display disruptive behaviors more frequently than their nonmigrant counterparts. Brief emergency interventions include safety planning, psychoeducation, parent training on communication and establishing routines, and behavioral therapies like activity scheduling and sleep hygiene.

Given the current political and climate crisis, the number of forcedly displaced individuals continues to rise, posing new challenges to host societies aiming to support and respond to the needs of those fleeing war or persecution. In this article, we turn our attention to current and historical sociopolitical contexts influencing the mental health of forcedly displaced children (ie, refugee, asylum-seeking, and undocumented) during their resettlement in high-income countries, proposing timely ways to respond to evolving needs and recommendations to redress ubiquitous structural inequities that act as barriers to education and care for the children, youth, and families seeking sanctuary.

Migration across the Americas is an ever-changing process with current trends including increased migration into the United States of Latine youth. Experiences before, during, and after migration can increase the risk of psychiatric illness, including discriminatory and exclusionary experiences when accessing care. Acculturation typically focuses on the process that the immigrant group experiences when coming into contact with a host culture. Members of the host culture and systems of care can take intentional steps to acculturate themselves in an integrative manner in an effort to reduce host–immigrant friction and better coordinate care across systems.

Refugee populations are diverse and can present with a variety of unique and complex circumstances. The purpose of this article is to examine an organization that provides care to refugee youth, the ways in which this is accomplished, and a few of the challenges that have been faced. Specifically, the work of this organization will be examined using a Systems of Care philosophy to demonstrate how using these concepts can assist in providing sensitive, high-quality care.

CHILD AND ADOLESCENT PSYCHIATRIC CLINICS

SERIES OF RELATED INTEREST
Psychiatric Clinics
https://www.psych.theclinics.com/
Pediatric Clinics
https://www.pediatric.theclinics.com/

THE CLINICS ARE AVAILABLE ONLINE!
Access your subscription at:
www.theclinics.com

Preface

Supporting the Mental Health of Migrant Children, Youth, and Families

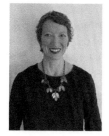
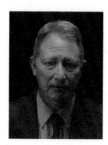
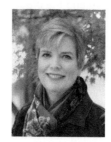

Margaret Cary, MD, MPH   Joshua D. Feder, MD   Alison Monds Ward, MD

Editors

> *My grandmother said that our 'Cadejos' guided us on the right path. When a baby is born, she receives a spirit animal to guide her, and they appear when they are most needed.*
> — *11-year-old girl from Guatemala (Sanchez and colleagues, "Cultural Considerations and Response to Trauma for Displaced Children at the Border," in this issue)*

Children, youth, and families who migrate to the United States are driven by need and carried by courage, determination, and resilience. The articles in this issue describe how mental health clinicians can be guided by the experiences, culturally based preferences, and requests of those who have migrated to best support their emotional well-being. Being humble, curious, and flexible, fostering connections, and participating in advocacy are foundational to the support.

In 2022, more than 152,000 migrant children were apprehended by the US border patrol, and nearly 130,000 entered the US shelter system.[1] These numbers have risen dramatically since the approximately 8000 apprehended in 2008. While most are teens, many are children, some very young, and some are young parents traveling with their own children.[1,2] The global numbers of migrant and refugee children and youth experiencing posttraumatic stress symptoms after arduous journeys and multiple traumatic events are as high as 54% per data obtained before the COVID-19 pandemic.[3] While US society experiences severe shortages of mental health services and providers, migrant and refugee children and families typically have significant barriers to accessing even more rare culturally and linguistically responsive care. As our communities become home for these children, many living without their parents, we

Child Adolesc Psychiatric Clin N Am 33 (2024) xiii–xv
https://doi.org/10.1016/j.chc.2023.10.001
1056-4993/24/© 2023 Published by Elsevier Inc.

will meet them in schools, community events, places of faith, clinics, emergency rooms, and hospitals. This collection introduces you to the common experiences of these children, youth, and families, describes the systems that impact them, gives you practical clinical advice, and offers a vision for care that we hope will inspire you.

The articles are organized to reflect the lived experiences, beginning with the migrant journey, cultural considerations for care, and observations of an American child psychiatrist working in Mexico. Next, the systemic context is described as well as our role in advocacy. Following this are best practices to treatment for the most common clinical presentations. This collection concludes with considerations for the phases of care and the practices and community-based systems that can impact well-being.

When we strengthen our competence and capacity to support and care for displaced children, youth, and families, we promote the well-being of our communities. The converse does not necessarily hold true. The unique premigration, migration, and postmigration journeys, acculturation stress, and legal precarity warrant tailored individual responses, community level supports, and system level advocacy.

We thank the contributors to this issue of *Child and Adolescent Psychiatric Clinics of North America*, who have shared their expertise in working with children, youth, and families who have migrated to the United States. They have summarized the historical context, detailed current practices, reviewed the extant literature, filled gaps in guidance, and encouraged us with actionable recommendations that will improve our clinical practices and our mental health systems. We are grateful for their time, work, and dedication. With this collection, they have contributed to ensuring the needs of displaced children and families are visible. This collection provides the guidance to promote the well-being of those who have migrated, now it is up to us to choose to contribute to the provision of care.

Margaret Cary, MD, MPH
Oregon Health Authority
Portland, OR 97232, USA

Yellowhawk Tribal Health Center

Joshua D. Feder, MD
Editor in Chief, the Carlat Child Psychiatry Report
Co-Chair, Disaster & Trauma Issues Committee, American Academy of Child &
Adolescent Psychiatry
Solana Beach, CA, USA

Alison Monds Ward, MD
Mental and Behavioral Health Services
Division of Health for Unaccompanied Children
Office of Refugee Resettlement
US Department of Health and Human Services

E-mail addresses:
margaret.cary@oha.oregon.gov (M. Cary)
jdfeder@mac.com (J.D. Feder)
alison.ward@acf.hhs.gov (A.M. Ward)

REFERENCES

1. Cheatham A, Roy D. US detention of child migrants. Center for Foreign Relations; 2023. Available at: https://www.cfr.org/backgrounder/us-detention-child-migrants. Accessed September 16, 2023.
2. Transactional Records Access Clearninghouse (TRAC). Growing number of children try to enter the U.S. Syracuse University; 2022. Available at: https://trac.syr.edu/immigration/reports/687/. Accessed September 16, 2023.
3. Frounfelker RL, Miconi D, Farrar J, et al. Mental health of refugee children and youth: epidemiology, interventions, and future directions. Annu Rev Public Health 2020;41: 159–76. https://doi.org/10.1146/annurev-publhealth-040119-094230. Epub 2020 Jan 7. PMID: 31910713; PMCID: PMC9307067.

Interview

Addressing Health Inequity and Mental Health of Migrant Children at the Border

Dr Joshua D. Feder Interviewing Dr Karina Anaya at Refugee Health Alliance

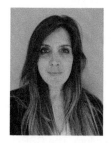   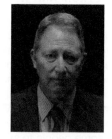

V. Karina Anaya, MD   Joshua D. Feder, MD

DR FEDER: TELL US ABOUT YOUR WORK WITH REFUGEE AND MIGRANT KIDS.

Dr Anaya: I trained with underserved populations at LA County and USC for both adult and child/adolescent psychiatry. The population I worked most closely with were immigrant families, LGBTQ youth, and their intersection. When I finished training, I started working with Refugee Health Alliance in Tijuana once to twice per month, providing free care for patients, supporting medical providers, and participating in advocacy. Both of my parents are immigrants, and luckily, Spanish was my first language, so I felt like I had some insight and skills that might be a good foundation for supporting humanitarian work at the border.

DR FEDER: DOES THIS CROSS-BORDER WORK REQUIRE A SPECIAL LICENSE?

Dr Anaya: Under Refugee Health Alliance (RHA), health care providers can volunteer to provide health care, under the supervision of a local Mexican physician. It's very difficult to get a Mexican medical license. To our knowledge, we are not aware of any other humanitarian aid organizations operating under any humanitarian license.

Child Adolesc Psychiatric Clin N Am 33 (2024) xvii–xxiii
https://doi.org/10.1016/j.chc.2023.10.006
1056-4993/24/© 2023 Published by Elsevier Inc.

DR FEDER: IS REFUGEE HEALTH ALLIANCE A VOLUNTEER ORGANIZATION?

Dr Anaya: RHA is a binational organization which strives to work as a nonhierarchical collective and a collaborative organization. Our policy is that US-based participants remain unpaid volunteers, while we employ Mexican citizens or migrants. It's necessary to sacrifice some privilege to participate in RHA, but it's also a privilege to participate in this way. We want the funds to go toward patient care, so we keep operations lean. We have a western medicine clinic, a midwifery practice, hygiene center, and a gender-affirming specialty clinic. Within our mental health branch, we have two psychiatrists who do remote consults from Mexico City, and one local Mexican psychiatrist who works part time. We have two staff psychologists and a small rotating team of volunteers who do remote therapeutic interventions and psychological first aid. On Saturdays, RHA organizes mobile clinic shelter visits, and many people from the US participate regularly.

DR FEDER: WHERE DO YOUR PATIENTS COME FROM AND WHAT IS THEIR IMMIGRATION STATUS?

Dr Anaya: Most are Mexican, or from the Northern Triangle countries, which are El Salvador, Honduras, or Guatemala. We have seen a large portion are from Haiti, but also Ukraine, Russia, Jamaica, Nicaragua, Venezuela, Cuba. During the pandemic, people had less mobility due to Title 42, fewer resources, and were more likely to be stuck at the border.[4] Title 42, which started during the Trump Administration, was extended during the Biden Administration, until it was finally rescinded in May 2023. Mexico has agreed to receive whoever the US expels. And now we have the new CBP-1 app, which is another frustrating barrier to allowing only some people to seek asylum. The CBP-1 app is like Ticketmaster for a place in line. But to use it you need to have secure access to the Internet, a smart phone to sign up for a meeting or a court date, and skin color which is easily recognizable by the facial recognition software of the app.

DR FEDER: DO YOU SEE CLIMATE CHANGE PLAYING A ROLE IN THEIR MIGRATION?

Dr Anaya: We don't consider climate refugees as a separate category from financial or political refugees. Climate change, which is the result of global neoliberal capital-market deregulation policies (such as privatizing industries and reducing state oversight), increases the frequency of natural disasters, making it harder for indigenous peoples to care for and live from their lands. The land is co-opted to serve the demands of the global market. We are seeing dominant white culture and racial capitalism leading to the loss of agricultural and economic instability for indigenous people. The political instability that imperialism inflicts often leads to local violence, gang culture, and corruption, and people become both economic and climate refugees.

DR FEDER: HOW DO YOU THINK THIS COMPARES WITH THE INEQUITIES WE SEE HERE IN THE US?

Dr Anaya: We can talk about so many different instances of inequities. However, people born on the US side of the border have so much more infrastructure in place to catch them, even though it seems like they don't, as well as the privilege to cross international borders. People south of the border without credentials, without insurance, without any money, don't have any kind of safety net to catch them. There aren't public hospitals where a child could be hospitalized. There are incredibly few child psychiatrists, and most of them are in private practice. It's been difficult to find anyone to help. The trauma that these children have experienced is mind-blowing. There are waves of people arriving with no access to food or water, no access to health care, turned away at hospitals, giving birth in front of the hospital because they are not granted access.

DR FEDER: HOW DO YOU CONCEPTUALIZE THE PREDICAMENT OF THESE PATIENTS IN YOUR PSYCHIATRIC WORK WITH THIS POPULATION?

Dr Anaya: We work toward health equity. The pathology I'm seeing is a result of inequitable distribution of resources due to neocolonialism and capitalism. Neocolonialism talks about how we've never left colonialism. We've just changed the face of it. France, the UK, and the United States still have commonwealth republics or territories with deep capitalistic expectations that affect territories' trade and their capacity to develop. I have seen how my psychiatric work with patients has shifted toward including discussions around the context in which their issues or "pathologies" are arising. I work from a radical healing framework and one rooted in liberation psychology[1] and antioppressive counseling,[2] meaning that I work with my clients toward acquiring critical consciousness, or a recognition of injustice and inequality. I do so knowing full well that the medications I offer are limited in their scope in this context, but moving toward radical hope and collectivism might prove as a support one day for their potentially revolutionary efforts.

DR FEDER: HOW DOES THIS RELATE TO CHILD AND ADOLESCENT PSYCHIATRY?

Dr Anaya: Western psychiatry uses race-based diagnostic tools that reinforce potentially racist notions that can harm our patients. In indigenous practice, the concept of wellness is often different.[3] It's not based on objective science but on subjective experiences of wellness and harmony with your body, your family, your community, and the earth, which are all considered a part of you, contributing to overall spiritual wellness. These concepts will be lost on us if we force people into western medicine ideologies. When we are working with children, we are often talking to them at a time when they are still developing their cultural or racial identity. Often, around ages of 6 to 10 years old they are becoming particularly savvy to injustices in their world. Our interventions with them have power to support their positive racial and cultural identification. When we validate their experiences of inequity, we are supporting them in their development of critical consciousness. The reason that developing critical consciousness is so important is that it can be protective from internalizing the oppression they experience, and personalizing the injustices they see.

DR FEDER: CAN YOU GIVE AN EXAMPLE OF A WESTERN PSYCHIATRIC CONCEPT THAT IS PROBLEMATIC IN AN INDIGENOUS SETTING?

Dr Anaya: Sure. The concept of ADHD is rooted in western European white supremacist ideals of performance and achievement. ADHD has so many strengths: you can be really in the moment, somatically based, great in an emergency, potentially great with your hands. All these things can be lost within the contextual framework of performance-driven western society. It's important to evaluate the context in which these pathologies are occurring. Is it society that's making it a problem? As another example, depression might be seen as a spiritual imbalance as well, being an imbalance in relation to one's ancestors or their family.

DR FEDER: WHAT DOES CHILD AND ADOLESCENT PSYCHIATRIC TREATMENT LOOK LIKE IN THIS SETTING?

Dr Anaya: We go to all the shelters, using strength-based and family-based interventions to create safety and routine in chaotic spaces. The psychologists I work with have been wonderful in reinforcing connection between parents and their children or building support groups within the clinic or shelter setting. I will interview parents and their children, review their cases, and determine if starting or continuing medication is appropriate. If a child is particularly psychologically vulnerable, at times I have been able to write humanitarian parole letters describing the necessity for allowing patients and their families to cross into the US to await their asylum court date instead of waiting on the border where free or low-cost mental health care is severely limited. Sometimes, I can write a letter describing my diagnostic impressions and recommendations for particular interventions that they can show their primary care provider when they land in the United States. Hopefully this will streamline their referral process once they arrive. Very often, parents will come to me with concerns for the instead of their changes in their child's behaviors since arriving to Tijuana after a long migratory passage. My role in those situations will look like providing education and support to the parents about what is considered a normal adjustment reaction and what more concerning signs of depression or anxiety might look like.

DR FEDER: DO YOU PRESCRIBE MEDICATIONS?

Dr Anaya: I do not prescribe there, but I consult with Mexican doctors who prescribe them. We have carefully crafted a formulary of psychiatric medications which would be considered safe to prescribe with a highly mobile population in which people are likely to discontinue them abruptly.

DR FEDER: HAVE YOU BEEN ABLE TO DO ANY KIND OF QUALITATIVE OR QUANTITATIVE STUDIES ON YOUR CARE?

Dr Anaya: We're protective of our patients. We don't want them to feel obligated to participate or worried that it'll affect the quality of their care, and they're always worried about being reported on. There are organizations that try to collect information. Most are legally oriented, but not everyone is going through legal pathways. So, we've been cautious about attempts at research through our organization. Physicians for Human Rights published a qualitative research study[1] on the mental health needs of the migrant population in Tijuana. The main findings were that over 90% of the population have significant psychiatric difficulties, largely trauma related. We would like to study our patients; however, for two years, I was the only psychiatrist going down to Tijuana. Now, we have grants to hire a few psychiatrists. So, we may be able to use qualitative approaches to look at outcomes.

DR FEDER: WHAT IS YOUR OBSERVATION OF THE ROLE OF BIGGER CHARITY ORGANIZATIONS IN ADDRESSING THE MENTAL HEALTH NEEDS OF THE REFUGEE POPULATION YOU ARE WORKING WITH?

Dr Anaya: Nonprofit charities say "let's go help poor people" within the context of capitalism. Nonprofit organizations are deeply nestled within capitalism and are doomed to perpetuate the marginalization of communities rather than working to address the root causes of inequities. Nonprofits allow the richest people in America to avoid paying taxes through tax-deductible donations, so instead of a strong social safety net that the government could be providing with taxes from the top 1%, marginalized communities are left with a patchwork of ineffective privatized services. Larger non-profits often have high administrative costs and become a tax shelter for donors, while framing what is considered an acceptable solution for societal issues (ie, homeless shelters as an appropriate solution rather than a restructured housing economy). RHA itself must try to keep this in mind, that it might also be in some ways perpetuating harm inadvertently.

DR FEDER: BASED ON YOUR EXPERIENCES, ARE THERE OTHER POLICY CHANGES THAT YOU BELIEVE COULD HELP THIS SITUATION?

Dr Anaya: Absolutely. Flexible border policies that respect people's rights to ask for protection if they face threat of life or freedom would significantly alter the landscape of human suffering that is piling up at the border towns of Mexico. This might look like efficient processing of personal data, alternatives to detention, which are often punitive, discriminatory, and inhumane, and appropriate staffing of the US immigration court system. Humanitarian organizations, such as RHA, try to effect change but can be seen as a bit of a Band-Aid if they're not also concurrently trying to work toward border abolition or abolition medicine.

DR FEDER: PLEASE GIVE US YOUR PERSPECTIVE ABOUT BORDER ABOLITION AND ABOLITION MEDICINE.

Dr Anaya: Border abolition is a scary term for some people. It's not knocking down all the walls but building a world where people can move from or stay in or return to their home. Most American citizens have the liberty to do that. Even though the border was closed, I could cross without any problems at all throughout the pandemic. Borders themselves are the infrastructural representation of structural violence like oppression or systemic racism. We can try to help folks by giving them antihypertensive medications or starting them on a sleep aid medication, but I'm not addressing the root causes unless I'm advocating to think about medical conditions critically. So, we can choose to continue practices that perpetuate structural racism, or we can dismantle them and rebuild just systems of care. Thinking about health inequity in a larger context helps you identify your own internal biases and helps you relate to your clients so that they can recognize your allyship, which I think furthers your capacity to be of service.

DR FEDER: WHAT ARE YOUR RECOMMENDATIONS ABOUT HOW CHILD AND ADOLESCENT PSYCHIATRISTS CAN HELP THIS POPULATION?

Dr Anaya: Child psychiatry made me a better adult psychiatrist because I understand trajectories a lot better, in terms of trauma, for example, along the spectrum from experiencing shame as a result of a critical caregiver to chronic sexual and physical abuse. This understanding helps me think about what I can accomplish with families living in an unsafe place. Migrant children are youth who have been uprooted, feeling lost and unstable, out of their routine and saddled with uncertainty. Talking about what trauma feels like can offer them a potential trajectory toward healing once they may get to a place that is more stable. I talk to them about learning how to feel safe and connected to your body again, and all the little ways we can do that. So, as a child psychiatrist, having words to explain that can be really helpful for this patient population.

DR FEDER: ARE THERE OTHER THINGS WE CAN DO?

Dr Anaya: Dedicate yourself to thinking critically about inequity and how we embody and project these dynamics onto our patients and how we may be participating in upholding systemic oppression through our job when we stay silent and fail to address the real causes of poor health. That's really important, no matter who you are or where you are. And on a more concrete level, you can also volunteer for organizations like Refugee Health Alliance (https://refugeehealthalliance.org/). Spending time on the ground is the best way to really gain an understanding of what is needed and how we can be of service. Or you can become an asylum evaluator. There's an online training program called Asylum Med Training that will help you learn to do sensitive, trauma-informed remote asylum evaluations (https://asylummedtraining.org/)

DR FEDER: WHAT ARE YOUR THOUGHTS ABOUT HOW THE BORDER SITUATION WILL PLAY OUT MOVING FORWARD?

Dr Anaya: The US Asylum system will continue to turn away asylum seekers, and Mexico has agreed to receive them indefinitely. The global climate crisis along with political unrest are inextricable and likely to continue to massively displace humans across the globe. Harsha Walia's book *Border and Rule*[5] really expertly draws the connections for us. But I see two paths moving forward. One path is to reimagine all of us as indigenous to our lands and to steward them, and each other. On the other path, we forget the indigenous world view, which for 40,000 years took care of and maintained its environmental beauty and protected rather than extracted its resources. The indigenous world view leans on a gift economy, treating the earth as a gift. *Braiding Sweetgrass*[6] is a beautiful book by Robin Wall Kimmerer, an indigenous plant biologist who talks through anecdotes, about how it's not the end of the world just yet, and we can reincorporate these worldviews to protect our land and our future.

Dr Feder: Thank you, Dr Anaya.

V. Karina Anaya, MD
Co-Director, Refugee Health Alliance

Joshua D. Feder, MD
Editor in Chief, the Carlat Child Psychiatry Report
Co-Chair, Disaster & Trauma Issues Committee, American Academy of Child &
Adolescent Psychiatry

E-mail addresses:
vkanaya@refugeehealthalliance.org (V.K. Anaya)
jdfeder@mac.com (J.D. Feder)

REFERENCES

1. Comas-Días L, Torres Rivera E. Liberation psychology: theory, method, practice, and social justice. Washington, DC: American Psychological Association; 2020.
2. Brown JD. Anti-oppressive counseling and psychotherapy. New York: Routledge; 2019.
3. Linklater R. Decolonizing trauma work: indigenous stories and strategies. Halifax: Fernwood Publishing; 2014.
4. Physicians for Human Rights. Neither safety nor health: how Title 42 expulsions harm health and violate rights. Asylum. 2012. Available at: https://phr.org/our-work/resources/neither-safety-nor-health/. Accessed September 16, 2023.

5. Walia H, Estes N. Border and rule: global migration, capitalism, and the rise of racist nationalism. Chicago: Haymarket Books; 2021.
6. Kimmerer R. Braiding sweetgrass: indigenous wisdom, scientific knowledge and the teachings of plants. Minneapolis: Milkweed Editns; 2015.

Upholding the Human Rights and Well-Being of Refugee Children Through Effective Clinical Care

Lisa R. Fortuna, MD, MPH[a],*, Michelle V. Porche, EdD[b]

KEYWORDS

- Refugee • Children • Trauma • Exploitation • Educational outcomes • Treatment
- Prevention • Families

KEY POINTS

- A refugee minor is a child or adolescent who has lost the protection of their country of origin, who has been forcibly displaced, and who cannot safely return home.
- There are a variety of reasons a child or adolescent and their family experience forced displacement, including facing the direct threat of violence resulting from conflict, targeted violence based on identity, and political violence.
- Stress related to cultural and social adaptation to a host country can negatively affect the psychological health of children, youth, and their families.
- Refugee children can face significant health-care and educational barriers in a resettlement country, and these should be addressed through systems of care, trauma focused and culturally responsive care approaches.

INTRODUCTION

Refugee children, adolescents and their families are a growing population globally. Based on United States law and the1951 Refugee Convention,[1] refugees are defined as "migrants seeking entry from a third country who are able to demonstrate that they have been persecuted, or have reason to fear persecution, on the basis of one of five protected grounds: race, religion, nationality, political opinion, or membership in a particular social group."[2] An important aspect of having a designation as a

[a] University of California Riverside, School of Medicine Education Building 2, 5th Floor, Psychiatry and Neurosciences, 900 University Avenue, Riverside, CA 92521, USA; [b] University of California, Psychiatry and Behavioral Sciences, 1001 Potrero Avenue, Building 5, 7M10, San Francisco, CA 94110, USA
* Corresponding author. University of California Riverside, School of Medicine Education Building 2, 5th Floor, Psychiatry and Neurosciences, 900 University Avenue, Riverside, CA 92521, USA
E-mail address: lisa.fortuna@medsch.ucr.edu

Child Adolesc Psychiatric Clin N Am 33 (2024) 111–124
https://doi.org/10.1016/j.chc.2023.09.003
childpsych.theclinics.com
1056-4993/24/© 2023 Elsevier Inc. All rights reserved.

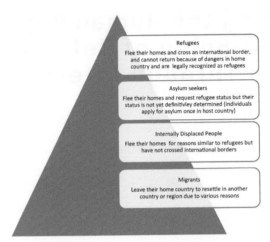

Fig. 1. Defining refugee, displaced people, asylum seekers, migrants.

refugee is experiencing forced displacement (**Fig. 1**), defined as migration that occurs because of persecution, armed conflict, generalized violence, or human rights violations.[3]

The United Nations 1951 Convention on the Status of Refugees is a legal code regarding the rights of refugees at an international level and it also defines under which conditions a person should be considered as a refugee and thus be given these rights. The Convention specifically provides protection to forcibly displaced persons who have experienced persecution or torture in their home countries and serves as the primary basis for refugee status determination internationally. However, some countries also use other refugee definitions, thus, can grant refugee status not based exclusively on persecution and can include other reasons for forced displacement. Increasingly, the term climate refugee is used for individuals experiencing forced displacement due to environmental disasters that have severely and negatively affected their home countries or region. Climate refugees are not included in the Convention definition of refugee; nonetheless, this group often faces traumatic experiences, poor health outcomes and need clinical and social services support. This can especially be the case for children, women, and families already living in poverty or those who are otherwise disenfranchised.[4]

More than 40% of refugees are children, and almost 1 in 3 children living outside their country of birth is a refugee person seeking safety.[5] These numbers encompass children whose refugee status has been formally confirmed and legally defined, as well as children in refugee-like situations (eg, children from Central America, Palestinian children in the West Bank or Gaza) who may or may not be fully recognized as a refugee based on international legal definitions.

Vulnerabilities and Trauma

The following are just some examples of the types of traumatic and violent situations that can lead to displacement for refugee children their families and communities.

- Sudanese refugee children witnessing traumatic events before departure from their home country, during attacks by the Sudanese military, that include instances of sexual violence, as well as of individuals being beaten, shot, bound, stabbed, strangled, drowned, and kidnapped.[6]

- Refugee children in Australia experiencing severe premigration traumas, including the lack of food, water, and shelter, forced separation from family members, murder of family or friends, kidnappings, sexual abuse, and torture.[7]
- Displaced unaccompanied child migrants from Central America fleeing some of the country's most violent cities.[8]

Regardless of legal status, forcibly displaced children face significant vulnerabilities throughout their journey, and these need to be of attention in trauma-informed and evidence-based care.

Vulnerabilities to exploitation and oppression

Refugee children, particularly those without documentation and those who travel alone, are vulnerable to abuse and exploitation. Examples of this include experiences of being trafficked and engaged in forced and exploited labor as minors.[9] Although many communities around the world have welcomed refugees, forcibly displaced children and their families often face discrimination and social marginalization in their home, in transit, and in the destination countries.[10] For example, destination countries often bar refugee children and their families from accessing education, health care, social protection, and other services that are available to the citizens of that nation. Many destination countries also lack intercultural support and policies for social integration. Because of these experiences, providers supporting refugee children and their families will need to consider the possible traumatic experiences and human rights violations that may need attention, including the need for legal protections and legal counsel.

Legal protections

The United Nations Convention on the Rights of the Child, the most widely ratified human rights treaty in history (although not by the United States), includes 4 articles that are particularly relevant to refugee children involved in or affected by forced displacement, which are as follows:

- The principle of nondiscrimination (Article 2) states that children have the right to not be discriminated against due to race, ethnicity, religion, or other identity.
- Best interests of the child (Article 3) states that children should be provided with the living situations, support and services that best promote their well-being, health, education, and relationships with their family and others.
- Right to life and survival and development (Article 6) includes the importance of education, shelter, and social support—among other supports for healthy development.

States Parties to the Convention are obliged to uphold its articles, regardless of a child's migration status. In 2015, Somalia ratified the Convention, bringing the total to 196 countries that have become States Parties to the Convention, leaving only the United States yet to ratify it.[11] Although the United States signed the treaty, it has not been ratified, and it is unlikely to receive the needed votes to do so in a divided Senate with polarized positions on child rearing and parochial education. Nonetheless, the protection of children, their well-being and development, rights regarding protection from human trafficking and involvement in armed conflict, are central principles for the care of refugee, migrant children in the United States and worldwide.

Displacement, Migration, and Trauma

There are several situations and circumstance that place refugee children at particular risk. These include human trafficking and exploitation, dangers in detention centers, and refugee camps. All these adverse events can be traumatic and contribute to poor mental health, including posttraumatic stress, anxiety, depression, and substance use disorders. Therefore, the assessment of refugee children and adolescents should include screening and identification of these experiences and the offering of evidence-based trauma treatment and social services and supports.

Trafficking occurs by definition when smugglers illegally move a migrant into another country, essentially a modern day slave trade that is a pervasive issue for children traveling both with and without their families.[12] In the United States, programs offer safe homes and treatment for trafficked young people, including vulnerable groups such as girls belonging to single-parent households, unaccompanied children, children from child-headed households, orphans, girls who were street traders, and girls whose mothers were street traders. Globally, girls aged younger than 18 years have been the main targets of sexual exploitation.[13] Although boys are also targets, the risk of sexual exploitation and abuse is higher for girls, and these experiences can have far-reaching effects on the physical and mental health. Children can also become victims of exploitation in their labor market, forced to work long hours, with minimum pay. Unaccompanied children may resort to dangerous jobs to send money back to their families of origin and to meet their own survival needs, rendering them at risk of labor exploitation.

Experiences of detention include when children are detained in prisons, military facilities, immigration detention centers, welfare centers, or educational facilities during the migration process. While detained, migrant children are often deprived of a range of rights, such as the right to physical and mental health care, privacy, education, and leisure.[14] Unfortunately, many countries do not have a legal time limit for detention of minors, leaving some children incarcerated or detained for indeterminate time periods. Some children are even detained together with adults and subjected to a harsher condition, treatment, and regimens. Such poor conditions have been the center of human rights litigation in the United States and globally, including the Flores Agreement in the United States,[15] which outlines the type of provisions of health care, education, and leisure children need to be provided. It also declares that a child or minor aged younger than 18 years should spend minimal time in detention and urges their expedient placement with family or other appropriate setting in the community.

Refugee camps are holding areas that can be found internationally and often operate at levels below acceptable standards of environmental health; overcrowding and a lack of wastewater networks and sanitation systems are common. Girls and sexual and gender minorities (eg, transwomen) at refugee camps may also be targeted and experience sexual assault.[16] Militia forces may also try to recruit and abduct children. With poor infrastructure and limited support services, refugee camps are often unable to protect children from these dangers.

Host Country Experiences (Postmigration)

Only a minority of refugees who travel into new host countries are allowed to start a new life there. Most refugees around the world are living in refugee camps or urban centers waiting to be able to return home.[3] For those who are starting a new life in a new country, there are 2 main options: seeking asylum or undergoing refugee resettlement.

Seeking asylum or special immigrant juvenile status

Asylum seekers are people who have formally applied for asylum once arriving in another country and who are still waiting for a decision on their status. In most situations, they need to apply for asylum within 1 year of arriving in the host country. Unaccompanied minors may face difficulties throughout the asylum process. Many children do not have the necessary documents for legal entry into a host country, leading them to avoid officials due to fear of being caught and deported to their home countries.[17] Without documented status, unaccompanied children often face challenges in acquiring education and health care in many countries. In the United States, once they have received a positive response on their application for asylum, they will obtain legal permanent residence in the United States. Special Immigrant Juvenile Status (SIJS) is an immigration classification available to certain undocumented immigrants aged younger than 21 years who can demonstrate that they have been abused, neglected, or abandoned by either one or both parents. Therefore, SIJS is another way for immigrant youth aged younger than 21 years to apply for and obtain legal permanent residence in the United States.

Refugee resettlement

Third country resettlement refers to the transfer of refugees from the country they have fled to another country that is more suitable to their needs and that has agreed to grant them permanent settlement. However, only a handful of nations prioritize this option and specifically consider children as a special category of refugees who are prioritized for resettlement.[18] The US Office of Refugee Resettlement currently works with state and local service providers to provide unaccompanied children with resettlement and foster care services. This service is guaranteed to unaccompanied refugee minors until they reach the age of majority or until they are reunited with vetted sponsors, which may be family or other adults identified by their families.

MENTAL HEALTH AND SYSTEMS OF CARE

Unaccompanied refugee children tend to display more behavioral problems and emotional distress than refugee children who have caretakers. Parental well-being plays a crucial role in enabling resettled refugees to transition into a new society. A child separated from caretakers during the process of resettlement faces an increased risk of developing a mental health problem,[19] including posttraumatic stress disorders. Distress may be further exacerbated by forced migration to a foreign country and the uncertain legal process of achieving refugee status protections or asylum determination. Migration and resettlement, particularly when these include separation from primary caregivers, are disruptive to development with potentially negative consequences for relational attachment and risk for internalizing and externalizing symptoms.[20] Research has shown that family reunification, formation of healthy social networks and supportive community connections, and provision of social services and professional support have contributed to successful resettlement of refugee children.[21] However, refugee children are particularly vulnerable to stigma regarding mental health problems before and during their resettlement.[22] Complicating matters, differences between parental and host country values and culture can create a rift between a refugee child and their family, make difficult their adaptation to a new society, and impede parental help seeking.

Caring for the mental health of refugee children must include attention to traumatic experiences, displacement, family trauma and separations, and address social support, educational needs, and community isolation. Additionally, mental health care should help promote cultural adaptation to host country and assist with overcoming barriers to care. **Table 1** identifies important examples of risk factors to address and protective factors that should be identified, assessed, and integrated into care planning to support strengths and promote well-being.

Table 1
Risk and protective factors for refugee child mental health

	Risk Factors	Protective Factors
Before travel	• Exposure to violent and potentially traumatic events • Torture • Poverty • History of mental health problems • Female, transgender, and nonbinary gender identity	• Higher educational attainment • Financially stable
During travel	• Exposure to violence and life-threatening events • Family separation • Human trafficking and exploitation • Female gender	• Direct route • Family support
During resettlement	• Food insecurity • Barriers to specialized care • Inadequate or poor living conditions • Uncertainty of asylum process	• Basic needs met • Quick asylum process • Legal support • Educational support • Emotionally supportive and regulating environments
Integration	• Social isolation • Unemployment • Discrimination • Acculturation stress • Family conflict • Downward social mobility	• Supportive social networks • Sense of belonging in host country • Ethnic identity and culturally supportive organizations including faith based

Overcoming Barriers to Care

There are many potential barriers to receiving mental health services. Structural and cultural factors can delay refugee children and their families from seeking medical and/or psychological help. Cultural barriers can include (not exhaustive) the following:

- Fear of discrimination and stigmatization
- Denial of mental illness as defined in the Western context
- Fear of the unknown consequences following diagnosis such as deportation, separation from family, and losing children
- Mistrust of Western biomedicine

There are also structural barriers to care, for example,

- Heightened instances of mental health complications in refugee populations for which providers have little training and may be inclined to overpathologize culturally bound symptoms or trauma symptoms.
- In the case of children, a lack of collateral information about previous behavioral health symptoms before the trauma of migration makes comprehensive care difficult.
- Time constraints: medical appointments are restricted to a small window of opportunity (specific and limited appointment schedules), making it difficult for facilitating engagement or even access to care.

Additionally, language and cultural differences can complicate a refugee's understanding of mental illness and mental health services.[23] Because children and adolescents have a greater capacity to adopt their host country's language and cultural practices, they are often used as intermediaries between service providers and their parents.[24] This may result in increased tension in family dynamics where culturally sensitive roles are reversed. Traditional family dynamics in refugee families disturbed by cultural adaptation tend to destabilize important cultural norms, which can create a rift between parent and child. These difficulties can cause an increased risk for depression, anxiety, and other mental health concerns in culturally adapted adolescent refugees. Relying on other family members or community members to relay clinical information has equally problematic results when they unintentionally exclude or include details relevant to comprehensive assessments and care planning.

Important strategies for overcoming barriers to care include practicing cultural humility, providing social supports, and including helpers such as community workers who can support and accompany families. This includes using the services of trained language interpreters[24] (which may be especially limited for some languages or dialects) and practicing family-driven care that may include their preference for consulting with religious leaders or organizations as intermediaries. Religious leaders are especially helpful especially when they can serve as cultural-religious brokers on topics related to trauma and mental health.

Program Case Example: Refugee Immigrant Assistance Center, Community Counseling Services

Refugee Immigrant Assistance Center (RIAC) Community Counseling is a community-based mental health and social support program created to serve the unique needs of refugees and immigrants. An important innovation of RIAC is that it is embedded in a refugee resettlement agency. This was planned intentionally, to improve access to services by offering a "one-stop" services approach. The clinic is staffed by multicultural and multilingual clinicians and case-managers, all who possess lived experience and professional expertise in refugee and immigrant mental health issues as well as a deep understanding of the cultural needs of the populations served. The program serves children and adults, and multigenerational families, providing resettlement services and case management and mental health services, and includes a psychiatrist, a nurse practitioner, and social workers. RIAC serves as a placement site for clinical internships for local psychology and social work schools, and they have academic partnerships with local universities, which additionally facilitates academic and research partnerships. For example, RIAC has served as a site for research on Trauma Systems Therapy for Refugee Youth. Clinical services include group therapy, individual therapy, psychopharmacology, and school-based consultations to support teachers and school counselors serving refugee students and families. There are specialized programs for men, women, and young adults, designed to address trauma, and age-specific and gender-specific concerns.

TREATMENT OPTIONS

The evidence-base for treatments that are specifically helpful for the youngest refugee children is limited. One evidence-based therapy for refugee families of infants and young children is Child-Parent Psychotherapy, an intervention model for children aged 0 to 5 years who have experienced traumatic events and has been extensively studied in culturally diverse families.[25] It integrates attachment, psychodynamic, developmental, trauma, social learning, and cognitive behavioral theories. Therapeutic sessions focus on supporting the relationship between a child and their caregiver to restore the child's cognitive, behavioral, and social functioning and include contextual factors that may affect the caregiver–child relationship (eg, cultural norms and socioeconomic and immigration-related stressors). Parent–Child Interaction Therapy (PCIT) is an evidence-based approach originally intended to treat disruptive behavior problems in children aged 2 to 7 years but in the last 40 years, it has been studied internationally and found to be an effective intervention for many behavioral and emotional issues including posttraumatic disorders.[26] PCIT includes supporting child-directed and parent-directed interactions. Therapists instruct and coach caregivers in play therapy and operant conditioning skills with the objective of encouraging warm, secure caregiver–child relationships.

Trauma-focused cognitive behavioral therapy (TF-CBT) was developed as an evidence-based treatment approach and is based on traditional cognitive behavioral therapy for traumatized children. It is a flexible component-based treatment model made up of both individual and joint child and parent sessions.[27,28] A meta-analysis[29] including 4 studies of TF-CBT provided evidence of TF-CBT's effectiveness in decreasing trauma symptoms and sustainment of these results during follow-up assessment among refugee children participants. However, the authors conclude that despite TF-CBT effectiveness for trauma symptoms treatment, there is still limited evidence to suggest that TF-CBT is effective for all refugee children due to the pilot nature of the studies, and its underutilization in traumatized refugee children from different cultural backgrounds. They called for future studies to be conducted TF-CBT interventions with diverse refugee children to provide more empirical support for its effectiveness.

Trauma Systems Therapy for Refugees (TST-R)[30–32] is a phase-based model of care that includes both individual and/or home-based support depending on the child's needs. TST interventions address both a child's self-regulation and social environment. In TST-R, services are often embedded in school systems to reduce barriers to seeking care based on evidence that refugee families are more likely to seek help in a school setting. Of note, cultural brokering, the inclusion of a cultural expert is an essential component of the TST-R model. A cultural broker is incorporated into each of the 4 tiers. The broadest level of care includes community engagement activities focused on developing trust between communities and providers and providing education about culture, mental health, and community needs. Throughout these activities, efforts are made to destigmatize mental health services and help seeking. The second level of care focuses on preventive skills-based groups for refugee youth that focus on increasing self-regulation skills, decreasing acculturative stress, and increasing social support, factors known to be associated with better mental health among refugee youth. The third and fourth levels of care focus on youth who demonstrate significant mental health needs and integrates emotional regulation and other cognitive behavioral therapy skills. Youth receive community-based, linguistically, and culturally sensitive care and families receive legal assistance and resettlement services as needed.

Education and School

Refugee children may experience disruptive schooling in their country of origin, or they may have received no formal education at all (UNHCR, 2022). Studies of migrant children globally found that experiences of discrimination in school negatively influence mental health.[10] In the United States, children's challenges in making up learning loss related to displacement is exacerbated by racial bias in the educational system and limited educator training in child mental health and behavioral responses that result from trauma.[33] Misunderstandings based on cultural beliefs and lack of trauma-informed training form the context of behavioral issues that teachers and school staff are not always well prepared to understand or to respond. Trauma can impede the ability to learn[34] and can cause fear toward people in positions of authority (such as teachers and principals).

High-quality education (evidence-based learning curriculum, well-trained instructors with documented qualifications, physical environment, higher teacher–student ratios) with inclusive practices (flexible and responsive to the local stakeholders) led by supportive teachers helps refugee children feel safe in the present, achieve success in school, and enables them to be productive in the future.[35,36] School dropout rates are highest for migrant children with a trauma history,[37] and they may also be influenced by self-perceptions of limited academic ability, othering from peers and educators, and/or a lack of educational preparation before entering the host-country school. Refugees may also experience school pushout in cases where educators are unprepared or unwilling to support the needs of migrant students.[38] There are several important cultural considerations for schools to think about in serving refugee children and their families, some examples include the following:

- Facilitating caregiver involvement: When caregiver involvement and support are lacking, a child's academic success decreases substantially. Refugee parents or guardians are often unable to help their children with homework due to language barriers. Caregivers often do not understand the concept of parent–teacher meetings and/or never expect to be a part of their child's education due to pre-existing cultural beliefs.
- Youth cultural assimilation: It can cause alienation of youth from their parents and country of origin and create barriers and tension between the parent and child.
- Antibullying interventions: Refugee youth face higher rates of bullying,[39] including social and individual rejection or hostile discrimination, which can cause additional trauma when refugee children are treated cruelly by their peers and adults. A review of antibullying interventions identified decreased internalizing symptoms,[40] and a clinical trial found that having peers of similar migrant backgrounds empowered vulnerable youth and decreased victimization.[41]
- Behavioral issues: They are caused by the adjustment issues and survival behaviors learned in refugee camps or during other adverse experiences and can create ongoing school problems if not identified and skillfully addressed in a trauma informed way. Within racially biased educational systems, clinical symptoms are too often simply interpreted as conduct problems.[33]

Curriculum Case Example for Supporting Educational Outcomes and Related Recommendations

In response to an intensive needs assessment of a refugee community in New England seeking to support children's well-being and academic success, a parent support intervention curriculum was codeveloped by the authors and community leaders from African countries and Bhutan.[42] The intervention was informed by a learning collaborative with the community and by results from interviews with youth, caregivers, mental health professionals, educators, law enforcement and justice agencies, social services workers, government officials, and clergy. Key education themes included the mismatch of expectations of parent involvement in US schools with more rigid boundaries for parental involvement in home countries, as well as limited confidence in helping with homework due to language and content barriers, and acculturation stress. Children who experienced trauma symptoms were unlikely to have teachers who accurately interpreted the meanings of their behaviors or knew how to respond. Most distressing for parents was that corporal punishment accepted in home countries would lead to social services reporting in US schools. Thus the

12-week parenting support intervention included modules that described expectations and policies of US schools and social service agencies, ways to support academic success that did not require content knowledge, alternative approaches to discipline, and strategies for family communication that incorporated attention to acculturative stress. For implementation of the intervention, a bilingual community liaison was hired to facilitate meetings between parents, teachers, and school counselors. Evaluation results showed improved behavioral and academic outcomes for the children and high satisfaction ratings from caregivers.[42]

Other recommendations for school success include the following:

- Course materials should be appropriate for the specific learning needs of refugee children and provide for a wide range of skills in order to give refugee children strong academic support.
- Educators should spend time with refugee families to assess previous educational experiences of the child and help to place the child in the correct grade level and to provide any necessary accommodations.
- Teachers in the United States often have little experience with the trauma that refugees often face. Therefore, educational resources and training for educators and school counselors can be helpful.
- Refugee children thrive in classroom environments where all students are valued and invited to share their cultural heritage. A sense of belonging and the ability to flourish and become part of the new host society are factors predicting the well-being of refugee children in academics.
- Extracurricular resources that can be provided to refugee children include supplementary curriculum enrichment resources that reflect their cultural values, videos in parental language on school awareness, informational leaflets, and handbooks, as well as trauma-informed resources that serve to benefit refugee youth and parental involvement in the school.
- School policies, expectations, and parent's rights should be translated into the parent's native language because many parents do not speak English proficiently.
- Educators need to understand the multiple demands placed on parents (such as work and family care) and be prepared to offer flexibility in meeting times with families. Parents have made the journey to a new country, along with many sacrifices, in hopes of providing opportunity for their child, so educators should not equate challenges in scheduling with lack of caring.

Accurate assessments for refugee children with disabilities are challenging given language barriers that can include limited interpreter options along with lack of cultural responsiveness[43] and a dearth of translated and validated disability assessments[44] and trauma and mental health screening tools[45] in languages other than English and Spanish. Improved assessments and services are critical for refugee children who are particularly vulnerable to physical and sexual abuse, exploitation, and neglect. Reassessment may also be required because initial assessments can result in underperformance due to hyperarousal, lack of exposure to standardized testing, and lack of limited educational opportunity as well as cultural mismatch between the child and the examiner. Children are not only often excluded from their education but also may not be provided the necessary supports for realizing and reaching their full potential.[46] In refugee camps and temporary shelters, and in schools within the countries they eventually resettle, the needs of refugee children with disabilities are often overlooked or difficult to address. Consultation from child mental health and educational professionals with experience and expertise in working with the special needs of refugee children with disabilities should be sought to ensure necessary support is provided.

SUMMARY

Refugee children in resettlement and their families have often faced significant traumatic experiences before migration and then must navigate the social and psychological stress of adapting to a new country. Forced displacement is increasing due to armed conflict and political violence, and more recently, influenced by climate change. Situations and circumstances premigration, during, and postmigration have significant influence on the mental health of refugee children. Although there are policies enacted within and between countries to protect children, there is variation in legislation and implementation in the United States and elsewhere across the globe. In addition to uneven protections, children and adolescents experience human trafficking and exploitation, and dangers in detention centers and refugee camps. All these adverse events can be traumatic and contribute to poor mental health, including posttraumatic, stress, anxiety, depression, and substance use disorders. Therefore, the assessment of refugee children and adolescents should include screening and identification of these experiences and the offering of evidence-based trauma treatment and social supports to promote their well-being and thriving.

CLINICS CARE POINTS

- Refugee experiences and mental health needs require screening for and addressing exposure to trauma and exploitation, with referral and provision of mental health services that offer cultural and linguistic access and expertise.

- Refugee mental health services for children necessitate comprehensive services, including medical, mental health, educational and social supports and case management, family supports including resettlement services, employment and housing, and legal services.

- Psychoeducation and evidence-based interventions for the children and caregivers can assist with intergenerational trauma and family well-being.

- Clinicians need to be proactive in improving mental health access and engagement strategies, including promoting approaches that use cultural humility, enhancing cultural awareness and sensitivity of mainstream providers, and facilitating ethnically matched professionals and paraprofessionals.

- Trauma-sensitive approaches emphasize helping school staff understand the influence of trauma on school functioning and seeing behavior through this lens; building trusting relationships among teachers and peers; helping students develop the ability to self-regulate behaviors, emotions, and attention; supporting student success in academic and nonacademic areas; and promoting physical and emotional health.

- Culturally responsive clinics and centers are well positioned to offer interventions designed to address trauma, reduce resettlement stress, and provide case management and preventive interventions that support child and family strengths.

DISCLOSURE

The authors have nothing to disclose.

REFERENCES

1. World Health Organization. International migration, health and human rights. Office of the high commissioner for human rights, . International Organization for Migration. Geneva Switzerland: World Health Organization; 2013.

2. American Immigration Council. An overview of U.S. refugee law and policy. 2022.
3. UNHCR. Global trends: Forced displacement in 2022.
4. Mahapatra B, Chaudhuri T, Saggurti N. Climate change vulnerability, and health of women and children: evidence from India using district level data. Int J Gynaecol Obstet 2023;160(2):437–46.
5. UNICEF. Child displacement. 2022.
6. Meyer SR, Yu G, Rieders E, et al. Child labor, sex and mental health outcomes amongst adolescent refugees. J Adolesc 2020;81:52–60.
7. Zwi K, Sealy L, Samir N, et al. Asylum seeking children and adolescents in Australian immigration detention on Nauru: a longitudinal cohort study. BMJ Paediatr Open 2020;4(1):e000615.
8. Sawyer CB, Márquez J. Senseless violence against Central American unaccompanied minors: historical background and call for help. J Psychol 2017;151(1): 69–75.
9. Arakelyan S, Ager A. Annual Research Review: a multilevel bioecological analysis of factors influencing the mental health and psychosocial well-being of refugee children. J Child Psychol Psychiatry 2021;62(5):484–509.
10. Metzner F, Adedeji A, Wichmann ML, et al. Experiences of discrimination and everyday racism among children and adolescents with an immigrant background - results of a systematic literature review on the impact of discrimination on the developmental outcomes of minors worldwide. Front Psychol 2022;13:805941.
11. United Nations. UN lauds Somalia as country ratifies landmark children's rights treaty. New York, NY: UN News; 2015.
12. Wood LCN. Child modern slavery, trafficking and health: a practical review of factors contributing to children's vulnerability and the potential impacts of severe exploitation on health. BMJ Paediatr Open 2020;4(1):e000327.
13. Stöckl H, Fabbri C, Cook H, et al. Human trafficking and violence: findings from the largest global dataset of trafficking survivors. J Migr Health 2021;4:100073.
14. Dudley M, Steel Z, Mares S, et al. Children and young people in immigration detention. Curr Opin Psychiatry 2012;25(4):285–92.
15. Roth BJ, Grace BL, Seay KD. Mechanisms of deterrence: federal immigration policies and the erosion of immigrant children's rights. Am J Public Health 2020; 110(1):84–6.
16. Tirado V, Chu J, Hanson C, et al. Barriers and facilitators for the sexual and reproductive health and rights of young people in refugee contexts globally: a scoping review. PLoS One 2020;15(7):e0236316.
17. Zayas LH, Brabeck KM, Heffron LC, et al. Charting directions for research on immigrant children affected by undocumented status. Hisp J Behav Sci 2017; 39(4):412–35.
18. Norwegian Refugee Council. A few countries take responsibility for most of the world's refugees. Olso, Norway: Norwegian Refugee Council; 2022.
19. Mares S. Mental health consequences of detaining children and families who seek asylum: a scoping review. Eur Child Adolesc Psychiatr 2021;30(10): 1615–39.
20. Cohodes EM, Kribakaran S, Odriozola P, et al. Migration-related trauma and mental health among migrant children emigrating from Mexico and Central America to the United States: effects on developmental neurobiology and implications for policy. Dev Psychobiol 2021;63(6):e22158.
21. Griswold KS, Vest BM, Lynch-Jiles A, et al. "I just need to be with my family": resettlement experiences of asylum seeker and refugee survivors of torture. Glob Health 2021;17(1):27.

22. Karamehic-Muratovic A, Sichling F, Doherty C. Perceptions of parents' mental health and perceived stigma by refugee youth in the U.S. context. Community Ment Health J 2022;58(8):1457–67.

23. Kim SY, Schwartz SJ, Perreira KM, et al. Culture's influence on stressors, parental socialization, and developmental processes in the mental health of children of immigrants. Annu Rev Clin Psychol 2018;14:343–70.

24. Clarke SK, Jaffe J, Mutch R. Overcoming communication barriers in refugee health care. Pediatr Clin 2019;66(3):669–86.

25. Ghosh Ippen C, Harris WW, Van Horn P, et al. Traumatic and stressful events in early childhood: can treatment help those at highest risk? Child Abuse Negl 2011;35(7):504–13.

26. Lieneman CC, Brabson LA, Highlander A, et al. Parent-child interaction therapy: current perspectives. Psychol Res Behav Manag 2017;10:239–56.

27. Cohen JA, Mannarino AP. Trauma-focused cognitive behavior therapy for traumatized children and families. Child Adolesc Psychiatr Clin N Am 2015;24(3):557–70.

28. Cohen JA, Mannarino AP, Deblinger E. Treating trauma and traumatic grief in children and adolescents. 2nd edition. New York, NY, US: Guilford Press; 2017.

29. Chipalo E. Is Trauma Focused-Cognitive Behavioral Therapy (TF-CBT) effective in reducing trauma symptoms among traumatized refugee children? A systematic review. J Child Adolesc Trauma 2021;14(4):545–58.

30. Benson MA, Abdi SM, Miller AB, et al. Trauma systems therapy for refugee children and families. In: Mental health of refugee and conflict-affected populations: theory, research and clinical practice. Cham, Switzerland: Springer Nature Switzerland AG; 2018. p. 243–59.

31. Ellis BH. Treating traumatized immigrant and refugee youth center for health and health care in schools. Washington, DC: Georgetown University; 2010.

32. Ellis BH. School-based trauma systems therapy for refugees: engaging partners. Atlanta, GA: The annual meeting of the international society for traumatic stress studies; 2009.

33. Dohrmann E, Porche MV, Ijadi-Maghsoodi R, et al. Racial disparities in the education system: opportunities for justice in schools. Child Adolesc Psychiatr Clin N Am 2022;31(2):193–209.

34. Malarbi S, Abu-Rayya HM, Muscara F, et al. Neuropsychological functioning of childhood trauma and post-traumatic stress disorder: a meta-analysis. Neurosci Biobehav Rev 2017;72:68–86.

35. Aghajafari F, Pianorosa E, Premji Z, et al. Academic achievement and psychosocial adjustment in child refugees: a systematic review. J Trauma Stress 2020;33(6):908–16.

36. Love HR, Horn E. Definition, context, quality: current issues in research examining high-quality inclusive education. Top Early Child Spec Educ 2019;40(4):204–16.

37. Porche MV, Fortuna LR, Lin J, et al. Childhood trauma and psychiatric disorders as correlates of school dropout in a national sample of young adults. Child Dev 2011;82(3):982–98.

38. Lukes M. Pushouts, shutouts, and holdouts: educational experiences of Latino immigrant young adults in New York City. Urban Educ 2013;49(7):806–34.

39. Pottie K, Dahal G, Georgiades K, et al. Do first generation immigrant adolescents face higher rates of bullying, violence and suicidal behaviours than do third generation and native born? J Immigr Minor Health 2015;17(5):1557–66.

40. Guzman-Holst C, Zaneva M, Chessell C, et al. Research Review: do antibullying interventions reduce internalizing symptoms? A systematic review, meta-analysis,

and meta-regression exploring intervention components, moderators, and mechanisms. J Child Psychol Psychiatry 2022;63(12):1454–65.

41. Zambuto V, Stefanelli F, Palladino BE, et al. The effect of the NoTrap! Antibullying program on ethnic victimization: when the peer educators' immigrant status matters. Dev Psychol 2022;58(6):1176–87.
42. Porche MV, Kirega G, Kayitesi C. Africans United for Stronger Families: development and pilot of a parent support program for resettled African refugees. Montreal, Canada: Biennial meeting of the Society for Research in Child Development; 2011.
43. McKay S. Immigrant children with special health care needs: a review. Curr Probl Pediatr Adolesc Health Care 2019;49(2):45–9.
44. Knuti Rodrigues K, Hambidge SJ, Dickinson M, et al. Developmental screening disparities for languages other than English and Spanish. Acad Pediatr 2016; 16(7):653–9.
45. Gadeberg AK, Montgomery E, Frederiksen HW, et al. Assessing trauma and mental health in refugee children and youth: a systematic review of validated screening and measurement tools. Eur J Public Health 2017;27(3):439–46.
46. Graham HR, Minhas RS, Paxton G. Learning problems in children of refugee background: a systematic review. Pediatrics 2016;137(6):e20153994.

Cultural Considerations and Response to Trauma for Displaced Children at the Border

Georgina Sanchez-Garcia, PhD[a],*, Beverly J. Bryant, MD[b],
Sarah L. Martin, MD[c]

KEYWORDS

- Migration • Displaced children • Trauma • Resilience • Cultural considerations

KEY POINTS

- The number of children and youths migrating from Central America and Mexico to the United States has drastically increased since the coronavirus disease 2019 pandemic.
- Children from these regions are diverse, including that Spanish may not be their first language. Although diverse, children share the right to grow in healthy conditions.
- Barriers to care can be formidable.
- Culturally modified, trauma-focused, evidence-based treatments are effective and possible.
- Strength and resilience must be emphasized over vulnerability or disease.

INTRODUCTION

Many children from Mexico and northern Central America are uprooted from their homes mainly due to poverty and violence that coexist and exacerbate each other.[1–11] The already dire conditions were untenable during and after the coronavirus disease 2019 (COVID-19) pandemic, further exposing inequity.[6,8,11] Mexico, El Salvador, Honduras, and Guatemala have the highest rates of child poverty in the Western Hemisphere, 51%, 44%, 70%, and 80%, respectively. Additionally, Central American children are 10 times more likely to be killed than children in the United States.[1,10–12]

In 2016, in El Salvador and Honduras, a child is a victim of homicide every day. In the same year in Guatemala, the number of violent deaths of children tripled. In 2017, 4 children died daily in Mexico because of violence. Girls often face additional violence, abuse, and discrimination related to the deep-rooted historical oppression of their gender.[10,11]

[a] The University of Texas at El Paso, 500 West University Avenue, El Paso, TX 79968, USA;
[b] Talkiatry, 4215 Lazy Creek Drive, Tyler, TX 75707, USA; [c] Texas Tech University Health Sciences Center, El Paso, 800 N. Mesa Street, El Paso, TX 79902, USA
* Corresponding author.
E-mail addresses: gsanchezgarci@utep.edu; ginauniversidad@gmail.com

Child Adolesc Psychiatric Clin N Am 33 (2024) 125–140
https://doi.org/10.1016/j.chc.2023.09.006
1056-4993/24/© 2023 Elsevier Inc. All rights reserved.

childpsych.theclinics.com

Furthermore, these countries have experienced devastating natural calamities, human trafficking, food scarcity, and illnesses.[1,3,4,7,10,11,13–17] In 2021, Mexican authorities registered 462,000 children migrating to the United States,[1,10,11] and nearly 150,000 were separated from their families.[1,14] The migration undertaken by the most disadvantaged children from these regions does so in conditions of extreme vulnerability.

Children zigzag across terrains and borders that have become increasingly restricted and dangerous.[6] Hungry and thirsty, with blisters on their feet, and having to sleep on the streets under the constant threat of criminal groups, some children manage to reach the United States but only to face new adversities waiting to be processed by US Customs and Border Protection. Those initial emotional impacts include separation from a trusted companion, depersonalization, and confinement in extreme cold. Subsequently, children may face other challenges, such as meeting a sponsor whom they do not know or being in foster care, learning another language, and acclimating to a new school system. These adverse experiences influence their psycho-emotional integrity, triggering emotions reflected at a cognitive, subjective, neurophysiological, and interactional level.[1–3,6,11,13,15,18]

Children separated from their families are at even greater risk of distress because they are exposed to the impactful experience of feeling alone in a threatening place. Distress tends to be contagious among migrant children residing together, which generates a constant state of alertness, further disrupting individual homeostasis.[4,11,19]

CULTURAL BACKGROUND

Significant differences exist between the countries' cultures in Mexico and northern Central America, as noted by the National Hispanic and Latino Mental Health Technology Transfer Care Network, funded by Substance Abuse and Mental Health Services Administration (SAMHSA).[20] Reports from *Instituto Nacional de Estadística, Geografía e Informática*[21] indicate that more than 80% of Mexicans identified as Catholic in 2021, whereas in the Northern Triangle, Evangelical identification has increased to ~ 40% and Catholic identification has reduced to ~ 33%.[21] This trend has implications for clinical practice because adult migrants may believe their suffering will be rewarded spiritually, whereas children may struggle to understand a supreme being (*Diosito*, as they call it) devoid of earthly justice. Thus, creating a safe space where they can express themselves freely is essential.[11]

Indigenous Peoples

In Mexico alone, more than 23 million people self-identify as indigenous, with 364 linguistic variations among the Nahuatl, Mayan, Zapotec, Mixtec, and Otomi indigenous groups.[13,22] The Northern Triangle and the South of Mexico share a significant sub-population of indigenous Mayans, with more than 6 million people belonging to 25 ethnic groups and 69 linguistic variations. Notably, between the years 1847 and 1937, intermittently, the Mayans stood against the landowners, direct descendants of the Spanish conquerors because they exploited them with impunity and were victims of all kinds of barbarity. After the forceful support of the government to the landowners, they did not submit to the oppressor, and many fled deep into the jungle of southern Mexico and Guatemala, where some survivors and descendants remained in small towns.[23]

Between 1960 and 1996, the indigenous Mayans of Guatemala faced a ruthless civil war because they fought against long-standing ethnic discrimination. In an attempt to maintain their dignity, they became the primary targets of government forces who used the army to launch a fierce counterinsurgency campaign. The war resulted in the death or disappearance of more than 200,000 Mayans, whereas another million indigenous people were displaced to Mexico. The violence committed against the indigenous Mayans during the civil war in Guatemala triggered a dynamic of emigration that continues to this day, especially given the country's high impunity rates.[11]

The previous paragraph is worth considering in clinical practice because children and other migrants from this region recognize what racism and oppression look like. Many experience the prevailing xenophobic discourse along the migration route and at their destination, feeling significantly humiliated and undermining trust in others. Additionally, their indigenous identity is often erased when children are miscategorized as Hispanic or Latino despite their language not being Spanish. Few interpreters speak native languages, generating relational barriers causing their isolation and harmful biopsychosocial consequences.[6,11,22]

Furthermore, according to the Council on Foreign Relations, in the fiscal year 2022, ~152,000 unaccompanied children arrived in the United States. In the same fiscal year, the Refugee Resettlement Office reported that 92% of unaccompanied migrant children came from the Northern Triangle and Mexico, with 15% aged younger than 12 years.[12] It is essential to consider the large number of indigenous children who are part of these percentages and who are most at risk due to the lack of knowledge about navigating the Westernized system and not having a trustworthy adult who can protect them and better explain their needs, including medical diagnosis.[6,11]

Indigenous peoples, migrating and already settled in the United States, identify as *some other* than Latinx or Hispanic.[22] They prefer their primary language to Spanish and rely on traditional practitioners for primary care.[20,22] According to the National Center on Cultural and Linguistic Responsiveness (US Department of Health and Human Services, 2018), many understand and treat diseases as cultural maladies classified as physical or spiritual.

Physical ailments, such as bone and muscular pain, skin conditions, and indigestion, are considered unforeseen and unintentional. However, maladies of the spirit affect the psyche and are often caused by people with malicious intentions. These include *mal de ojo* (evil eye), *susto* (an intense fright), and *Tiricia* (sadness of the soul).[22,24]

Indigenous peoples rely on traditional healers such as *Yerbero/a* (herbalists), *Sobador/a* (massage practitioners) (**Fig. 1**), *Huesero* (bone and muscle therapists), and *Curandera/o* (folk healers).[22] In the Maya community, it is essential to identify and

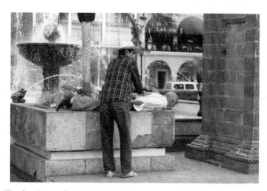

Fig. 1. *Sobador* in Tepic, Nayarit Mexico town square. (*Photo by* Beverly Bryant).

collaborate with individuals such as *Ajq'ijbab* (Mayan priest), Catholic priests, and other traditional authorities.[11,16]

Evidence-based treatments must recognize the importance of maintaining cultural rituals and traditions while focusing on strength and resilience rather than disease and vulnerability. Effective clinical care requires cultural humility, which involves self-reflection and self-criticism, by which one not only learns about another's culture but also begins by examining one's beliefs, cultural identity, and biases. Thus, with a more genuine and sensitive approach to the child's suffering, the clinician can work to restore trust and develop rapport.[25]

THE CHILDREN'S NARRATIVES

Sanchez-Garcia and Lusk interviewed 34 girls and 42 boys aged 8 to 12 years from Mexico and Central America at two strategic points, the Guatemala/Mexico border, and the Mexico/US border. They listened to their stories and assessed exposure to adverse events, traumatic stress (Child PTSD Symptom Scale), and childhood resilience (Child and Youth Resilience Measure).[7,10,11]

Children described their experiences using legends, family stories, and drawings.[6,7,10,11] The main reasons for leaving home were oppression, poverty, violence, climate change, and environmental calamities. Paradoxically, they showed remarkable resilience due to factors associated with cultural and social support, family, and faith.[6,7,10,11] Children's narratives can be viewed in the YouTube documentary: Exploring Resilience Among Migrant Children from Central America and Mexico En Route to the United States.[10]

The traumatic events that they experienced were as follows: hunger (33%), death threats (22%), witnessing a homicide of a family member or someone in the community (18%), walking for hours in unknown territories and the jungle at night (18%), thirst (17%), extortion by authorities (13%), physical and psychological abuse by child's father (13%), death of a family member due to COVID-19 (13%), and (at 9% each) witnessing the beating of one's parents, threatened conscription into a criminal gang, and xenophobia.[11] Although of lower percentages, the children also experienced feeling suffocated in trucks for hours, armed crossfire, rape, theft, and kidnapping (**Fig. 2**). Some spoke of the fear of the "polleros" or "coyotes" who were paid to get them over the border. Some had to escape, and others described being abandoned in the jungle.[6,8,10,11]

Of the 76 participants, 73.7% reported PTSD clinical symptoms, 40.8% severe.[11] Despite this, themes of resilience emerged involving family (parents, siblings, and grandparents); faith (Diosito, Jesus, Virgen de Guadalupe, and Nature Spirits);

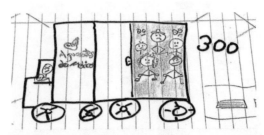

Fig. 2. *Polleros.* "The '*polleras*' put us on a covered truck. (...) We were 300 people." A 10-year-old boy from Guatemala. (*Adapted with permission from* Sanchez G. Trauma and Resilience among Migrant Children from Mexico and the Northern Triangle Enroute to the United States. Doctoral Thesis. 2022.)

character (integrity, courage, and perseverance); and relational health (interaction, play, camaraderie, and culture).[7,10,11]

Children's manifestations contained more suffering than psychiatric disorders. However, specific traumatic symptoms were also identified, significantly more severe in those migrating during extended periods, including stays in border shelters. Correlational, their resiliency resources diminished. Hence, timely interventions are of critical importance.[11,18]

BARRIERS TO CARE

Although Mexican and Central American young people living in the United States experience higher trauma rates than their White peers, they have limited access to mental health care and are more likely to end treatment prematurely due to barriers such as language resources, transportation, and lack of health insurance.[14,17] These barriers are even more significant for migrant children and youth seeking refuge.

As mentioned early, Spanish is not the primary language for many indigenous children and youths.[3,5,11,26] Finding translators who are not also family or friends can be difficult. Girls may be particularly reluctant to discuss details of their experiences in front of relatives, friends, or even male providers.[26] In addition, there is an ongoing fear of deportation after risking their lives to travel so far.[4,5]

Mental health interviews are not always confidential, and information obtained can be subpoenaed and used to discredit the individuals being interviewed or even their families and friends.[1,4,9,26] For example, instead of recording that "3 people entered the room," it is better to say that "several people entered the room." Moreover, it is better to say "sometime in the spring" than to record a specific date.[1]

Similarly, if children are encouraged to express their true feelings, such as saying, "I was so mad I felt like hitting a wall," that can be interpreted as having a history of violent behavior. If a child names a relative in the United States to be reunified, authorities can investigate that relative and deport them if their status is undocumented. Migrant children know it can be dangerous to communicate openly with mental health professionals.[1]

Moreover, the therapeutic intervention has to accompany the efforts of the people in the preventive fight against the causes of oppression, poverty, and violence and prioritize the defense of children's rights. In pursuing social justice, mental health professionals can play a significant role in advocating for the rights of migrant children at risk of suffering a preventable disorder or even death. By doing so, clinicians can elevate the dignity of their profession.[6,11]

CULTURALLY MODIFIED EVIDENCE-BASED TREATMENT

Judy Cohen and collaborators[16] studied CBT to treat trauma and traumatic grief in refugee youth, a review of which is available in Child and Adolescent Psychiatric Clinics of North America, July (2008). They emphasized that basic needs must be met before trauma-focused treatment can begin. Refugee and migrant populations often require medical, legal, occupational, and social services on arrival in the host country.[1,16] The first step must be establishing physical safety and psychological first aid.[1]

CULTURALLY MODIFIED TRAUMA-FOCUSED COGNITIVE BEHAVIORAL THERAPY

Cohen's group also developed culturally modified trauma-focused cognitive behavioral therapy (CM-TF-CBT) to provide evidence-based treatment to specific populations.[14,16] A comprehensive review can be found in the chapter, "Children of Latino

Descent: Culturally Modified TF-CBT" by de Arrellano and colleagues in *Trauma-Focused CBT for Children and Adolescents: Treatment Applications*.[14] In 2020, her group studied the feasibility and efficacy of implementing CM-TF-CBT for trauma-exposed youth in El Salvador. The project trained 15 Salvadoran psychologists in TF-CBT. They treated 121 children and adolescents in community-based settings and found it effective for reducing self-reported symptoms of trauma (Cohen's d = 2.04), depression (Cohen's d = 1.68), and anxiety (Cohen's d = 1.67).[18,27]

CM-TF-CBT recognizes cultural identity and the importance of maintaining cultural rituals and traditions while focusing on strength and resilience rather than illness. It integrates traditional values such as family (*la familia*), spirituality (*espiritualidad*), personalism (*personalismo*), respect (*respeto*), courage (*coraje, valentía*), and gender roles.[2,28] The use of "*cuentos*" (short stories) and "*dichos*" (proverbs) are important for cognitive restructuring,[2,19,28] especially for adolescents who may be adapted to collective analog thinking. Children in middle childhood often rely on empirical evidence.[11] TF-CBT transformers (*pasos para sanar*) (**Fig. 3**) are used during treatment and are culturally modified.[2,28,29] Several webinars are available online.[30,31]

CONTACT AND ENGAGE

A "Psychological First Aid for Displaced Persons" guide can be found on the National Child Traumatic Stress Network (NCTSN) website at NCTSN.org.[9,31] The first contact with a displaced child may include the following.[11,31]

- Sit or kneel to meet the child's eye level and speak in simple terms.
- Introduce yourself and clarify that you are a health provider and not responsible for immigration decisions.
- Consider your vocal tone and body language. Nonverbal cues can have a greater influence than words when someone feels threatened.
- Use open-ended questions to confirm their understanding because they may nod or signal agreement out of respect even if they do not fully understand.
- Ask the child about their pressing needs. Those needs may be more painful at that particular time than the main traumatic event.
- Ensure you have time to learn about them (eg, their name and something they want you to know about them, including cultural practices important to them).

Displaced children undergoing clinical consultations have likely experienced chronic stress. According to Dr Stephen Porges, founding director of the Traumatic Stress Consortium at the Kinsey Institute (cited by Sanchez-Garcia[11]), continual exposure to threats can be metabolically taxing and disrupt crucial neural systems in the

CM-TF-CBT Transformers	Pasos para Sanar
Learning about the trauma	Aprender sobre el trauma
Handling the stress	Manejar estress
Identifying and expressing feelings	Identificar y expresar emociones
Changing thoughts	Cambiando los pensamientos
Creating the trauma narrative	Creando la historia sobre el trauma
Working through	Procesar
Completion	Completar

Fig. 3. CM-TF-CBT transformers. (Echevarría Velez IS. Trauma-Focused Cognitive Behavioral Therapy: A Culturally-Modified Therapy to Work with Latino Children and Youths. National Hispanic and Latino Mental Health Technology Transfer Center. Published October 6, 2020. Accessed January 8, 2022. https://mhttcnetwork.org.)

brainstem necessary for survival; such disruption is expressed through the autonomic nervous system mechanisms, fight, flight, and, most likely in clinical settings, freeze. Not only is it critical to eliminate the stressor but it is also necessary to repair homeostatic functions involving the endocrine, limbic, and autonomic nervous systems.[11,18] Therefore, the process of self-regulation must first be promoted so the child can recognize that the threat is no longer there. An initial and effective way to promote the self-regulation process with displaced children is through spontaneous and active play, such as tag, mouse hunt, pillowcase races, or soccer. In this way, and with the clinician's competence to use safety signals such as facial expressions and tone of voice, the child will gradually recognize that they are in a safe place. As a result, children will be more able to develop rapport with the health provider.[11] Critically to consider is not using exposure therapy in the context of ongoing trauma.[1]

RESILIENCE RESOURCES

We define resilience as the child's ability to navigate their immediate social ecology to access resources and respond effectively to significant adversity.[6,7,11]

Family (La Familia)

Family connections are of the utmost importance. In her narrative, an 8-year-old girl from Honduras explained, "When we suffer, my family and I hug each other, we love each other, and we always try to be together" (**Fig. 4**). An 8-year-old child from El Salvador said, "I don't want to die from COVID-19 and go to heaven without my family. What am I going to do there alone? (**Fig. 5**).[6,7,10,11]

Family members need to be included in the treatment process.[2,28,29] De Arellano recommends assessing those directly and indirectly involved in the child's life and being willing to incorporate other family members into the treatment, especially fathers. Family members should also be involved in the planning and completion. It may be necessary to differentiate the child's needs when they seem to conflict with the family's needs.

Personalism (Personalismo)

Warm interpersonal connections are also meaningful, especially in developing trust.[2,28,29] The therapist may need to be prepared to use self-disclosure judiciously.

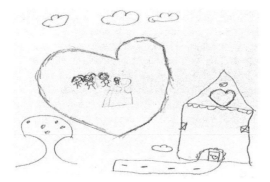

Fig. 4. *La Familia.* "When we suffer, my family and I hug each other, we love each other, and we always try to be together." An 8-year-old girl from Honduras. (*Adapted with permission from* Sanchez G. Trauma and Resilience among Migrant Children from Mexico and the Northern Triangle Enroute to the United States. Doctoral Thesis. 2022.)

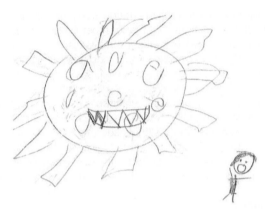

Fig. 5. COVID-19. "I don't want to die from COVID and go to heaven without my family. What am I going to do there alone?" An 8 year-old boy from El Salvador. (*Adapted with permission from* Sanchez G. Trauma and Resilience among Migrant Children from Mexico and the Northern Triangle Enroute to the United States. Doctoral Thesis. 2022.)

Boundaries need to be relaxed regarding accepting food and other small gifts. Flexibility when ending therapy sessions is also necessary.

Families may be reluctant to discuss their challenges outside the family[2,28] and *personalismo* can help to foster the trust necessary for sharing personal difficulties. The reluctance may be due to experiences of oppression, including from health-care systems. Their countries of origin often lack accessibility to health care for disadvantaged populations and provide impersonalized treatment when available. Clinicians must recognize the perceptions that they represent for the child and their caregivers.

One effective practice for establishing rapport is by directly introducing oneself to the head of the family and asking for their assistance in gathering all members in a circle to get to know them as a *familia*. It is important to allow the parent to lead the introductions. By doing so, the health provider facilitates the parent to show their leadership to their family, and therefore, their ability to protect them despite the current crisis they may be facing. This also exhibits the clinician's cultural competence by respecting the role of the parent within the family and may also initiate a subtle yet profound process: the parent's awareness of their human dignity. The health-care provider can ask if the family wants to express any salient concern before the individual session begins. Often, families will have pressing issues such as unmet basic needs or feelings of sadness from being separated from loved ones. From a genuine stand, the health provider can gesture solidarity with them by providing relevant information or simply saying, "I'm sorry to hear you're going through this." Children will observe that the health provider values their family and their ways, just as someone from their community would. This approach of *respeto*, along with *personalismo*, can help to foster trust for sharing personal difficulties.

Respect (Respeto)

Respect for the family roles of both adults and children is essential. Caregivers may need to permit children to discuss adult topics in therapy. The therapist must be careful not to put the child or a family member in a position to disagree with an authority figure, including the therapist.[2,28,29] Parents may believe that children should obey them simply out of respect. Parenting interventions such as praise or positive reinforcement may need to be framed as techniques for increasing respect rather than compliance.[2,28]

GENDER ROLES

In Mexican and Central American cultures, roles are evident in the family. Some women are still seen as submissive, self-sacrificing, and dependent; for many girls, this is the role model they are presented with. However, men are seen as providers and are expected to defend and protect the family.[14,29]

In 2020, of the 16.2 million migrants from Central America and Mexico, 48.7% were women and girls who faced challenges at all stages of the journey. The confluence of gender, age, ethnicity, nationality, and lack of documentation can lead to extreme human rights violations, including sexual abuse. Specifically, girls comprise the highest group of victims in organizations dedicated to human trafficking, which is why they are among the most at risk for trauma.[8]

Spirituality (Espiritualidad)

Spirituality and faith are significant sources of strength and healing. Children have often seen their families pray for divine intervention along their perilous journeys.[6,7,10,11] Children from Dr Sanchez-Garcia's study report:

"God always goes anywhere we go. All people have God to take care of them." An 8-year-old boy from El Salvador

*"The Virgen (sic) is a good person. She appeared to my cousin praying in the desert of Juarez and Texas. That is why we are going to cross there. The Guadalupana's smile is so pretty (**Fig. 6**)." A 12-year-old boy from Mexico.*

*"My grandmother said that our 'Cadejos' guided us on the right path. When a baby is born, she receives a spirit animal to guide her, and they appear when most needed (**Fig. 7**)." An 11-year-old girl from Guatemala.*

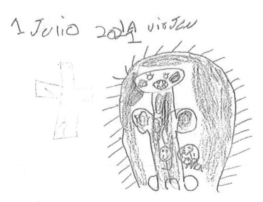

Fig. 6. The Virgin Mary. "The Virgin (sic) is a good person. She appeared to my cousin praying in the desert of Juarez and Texas. That is why we are going to cross there (...) The Guadalupana's smile is so pretty." A 12-year-old boy from Mexico. (*Adapted with permission from* Sanchez G. Trauma and Resilience among Migrant Children from Mexico and the Northern Triangle Enroute to the United States. Doctoral Thesis. 2022.)

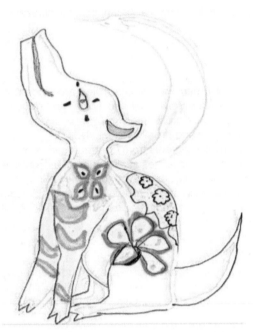

Fig. 7. Spirit Animals. "My grandmother said that our 'Cadejos' guided us on the right path. When a baby is born, she receives a spirit animal to guide her, and they appear when they are most needed." An 11-year-old girl from Guatemala. (*Adapted with permission from* Sanchez G. Trauma and Resilience among Migrant Children from Mexico and the Northern Triangle Enroute to the United States. Doctoral Thesis. 2022.)

"The Guatemalan Immigration agents did not let us cross. We had to walk through the jungle and cross the Paz River on a raft at night. It started to rain, the thunders (sic) didn't stop, and I was terrified of dying. Shortly after, the rain stopped, and we realized we had been next to the dock all that time. We had already arrived, and we hadn't realized it!"[10,11] An 11-year-old boy from El Salvador.

Courage (Coraje/Valentía)

Courage is a tenacious decision that implies an effort of body, mind, spirit, and zest. The term also includes discontent with a fatalistic idea.[32] A courageous person does not settle for what they perceive as unjust and, consequently, acts despite their fears. A 12-year-old boy from Mexico states, "Mentalize that you are going to suffer and that later it will be better. Control your emotions." (**Fig. 8**).[10,11] Although this can aid in resilience, it may also have to be overcome as a treatment barrier. This is where the use of a "*dicho*" (see **Fig. 1**) or proverb may be beneficial: "*Dios aprieta pero no ahorca*" (God squeezes but does not choke).[28]

Dichos (proverbs)

Dichos are sayings or proverbs that often convey traditional wisdom (**Fig. 9**).[19,33–36] Sayings such as "*Amor de madre, ni la nieve le hace enfriarse.* (Not even the snow, makes a mother's love cold) can be helpful when working with the TF-CBT Transformers or "*pasos para sanar*"[29] (see **Fig. 3**).

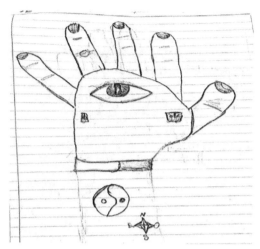

Fig. 8. Courage *(Coraje/Valentía)*. "Mentalize that you are going to suffer and that later it will be better. Control your emotions." A 12-year-old boy from Mexico. (*Adapted with permission from* Sanchez G. Trauma and Resilience among Migrant Children from Mexico and the Northern Triangle Enroute to the United States. Doctoral Thesis. 2022.)

Cuentos

Cuentos are short stories that often contain a life lesson, similar to a fable. Examples are the story of the "Little Red Ant" and "The Laughing Skull."[2,28] The following is an excerpt from De Arellano's chapter.[2]

Cuento of the Little Red Ant

There once was an ant that was smaller than everyone else, and thus believed she was weaker and different. One day she came across a piece of cake that she really wanted to bring home for her family to eat. She did not believe she could carry this cake by herself, and when she came across many other animals, she asked them to help her. However, no one could help her. In the end, she told herself to at least try to carry the cake before giving up, and it ended up that she could carry it all by herself after all!

In this excerpt, the value of *la familia* is clear. De Arellano points out that "by changing her thoughts," the little ant "gained confidence and learned she was capable of much more than she thought." Another excerpt from de Arellano's chapter.[2]

Cuento of the Laughing Skull

A long time ago, next to the convent of Santo Domingo, a skull sat in a niche in a wall. People would always pass by this skull but no one noticed it. One night, guards walking by heard noises, and suddenly the skull was floating, shaking, and screaming.

El que es buen gallo dondequiera canta	A good rooster can crow anywhere
Al burn entendedor pocas palabras	A good listener needs few words
Despues de la Lluvia sale el sol	After the rain comes the sun
Donde hay gana hay maña	Where there's a will there's a way

Fig. 9. *Dichos.* (*Adapted from* Gonzalez R, Ruiz A. *Mi Primer Libro de Dichos.* Children's Book Press; 1995 and Sellers JM. Folk Wisdom of Mexico. Chronicle Books; 2005.)

This happened many nights in a row until one of the guards finally decided to look closer at the skull, despite being very scared. As he approached, the skull fell to the ground, and the guards quickly learned that mice, which had built their home under the skull, were causing all the noise and movement.

Clearly, by confronting their fears, the guards gained significant knowledge and mastery over the situation. De Arellano states, "The message is that challenging one's thoughts, or the meanings attached to certain situations, can help improve feelings (eg, change fear to courage to relief) and behaviors."[2]

Clinical Vignettes

The resilience resources of children that have immigrated alone are astonishing. They are living examples of the *dicho* "*Dios ayuda a los que se ayudan*" (God helps those who help themselves). A 14-year-old girl who developed depression and anxiety that led to suicidal ideation on arrival to the United States shared her story while hospitalized. She and her 10-year-old brother were in extreme danger in Guatemala, escaping rather than simply surviving and staying home, enduring the dangerous overland route to the United States, and they walked thousands of miles in search of a better life. After crossing, they turned themselves into the nearest US Border Patrol Station to begin the process of obtaining a refugee visa. The girl became overwhelmed on reaching the safety of the foster care facility, where many unaccompanied children are placed if they do not have a family with whom they can be reunited. Despite the safety of the foster care facility, and being with other children in similar circumstances, the girl felt uncertainty, anxiety, and intolerable fear in this environment so different from her culture. She developed suicidal thoughts and was hospitalized. On the first day of hospitalization, she was hopeless and exhausted.

On the second day, she expressed feeling well and stated that she needed to return to the foster care facility as soon as possible to care for her brother. *Coraje* was a core value for this Guatemalan girl. The strength and intensity of her bravery overcame her fear and suffering, reflecting the proverb, "*Ante la adversidad. Calma!*" (In the face of adversity. Be calm!).

The previous case led us to reflect that concepts matter.[25] The word *migration*, either legal or illegal, that authorities and some health providers understand and use is very different or nonexistent for those who flee oppression, violence, and foreseen premature death and must find a route to survive. The violence that many displaced children are exposed to is, at times, beyond comprehension.

A 13-year-old boy was admitted to our inpatient unit for suicidal ideation. In his hometown in El Salvador, his father had been targeted by the local gang for his refusal to join. Soon after, his head was delivered to his family by mail. The remaining family members pooled their resources and hired a smuggler to take him to the United States. After reaching safety, he let his guard down, his suicidal ideation was identified, and he was transferred from the foster care facility to inpatient psychiatry. Maintaining composure while hearing this boy's story was a challenge for even the most experienced clinician but witnessing how quickly he recovered and became hopeful for the future was inspiring. While on the inpatient psychiatry unit, his biological mother was located, her background check was completed, and the approval was received for reunification. He was very excited to see her.

La familia was central to this child's recovery. His internal sense of *family* allowed him to keep the hope of seeing his mother, who emigrated shortly after his birth. After his acute recovery from the traumatic death of his father, the boy could not wait to be reunited with her in *El Norte*. The medical team recognized that the child emigrated unaccompanied, without family support. Aware of the child's plight, the medical team not only provided effective care but did so with compassion and sensitivity. Family support and humane medical treatment contributed to his emotional balance. Thus, the ecology surrounding a child makes a critical difference.[11]

Another example of a child over adversity involves a 7-year-old girl. A group of immigrants crossed the border aided by a human smuggler but the Border Patrol spotted them shortly after entering the United States. The group scattered to avoid being detained. Everyone escaped except the 7-year-old girl. She had been traveling with her father but he disappeared into the desert with the other traveling group members. She was brought to the Border Patrol station to be assessed for placement and to start the immigration process.

Despite being alone with strangers, she remained composed and showed no signs of panic or distress. She calmly looked around and assessed her options. She approached the nearest agent and asked him if he was the boss. When he replied in the affirmative, she said, "Good, I will just go home with you, and you can take care of me." She then proceeded to color with the crayons and paper he provided her. Before her transfer to the foster care facility, she proudly displayed her drawings to the agent and gave them to him as a gift. They were beautiful drawings full of color.

This young child personified the value of *personalismo* with her ability to connect with a stranger with a gift and a smile. The way she navigated the situation and her resilient resources was astounding. Even though her father abandoned her in a foreign country, she immediately switched gears and negotiated her survival. However, how long will her resilience last without our protection? Our involvement should not be only as a member of the medical profession but also as part of a society aware of its responsibility toward a child.

SUMMARY

Culturally modified evidence-based treatment is possible. The values of family, spirituality, character, and personalism enhance children's resilience. However, it is essential to recognize that displaced children come from diverse cultural backgrounds, and are in different developmental stages. Within their heterogeneity, children share the right to grow in an environment conducive to developing their full potential. Their humanitarian struggle shows resilient children who, without timely intervention, are exposed to complex trauma due to the intensity, chronicity, and complexity of their migration experience under inhumane conditions.

CLINICS CARE POINTS

- People migrating from Mexico and northern Central America are diverse and heterogenous.[22]

- Care must be given to distinguish among groups, and providers must be mindful that Spanish is neither the primary language for many indigenous children nor is Catholicism or Evangelicalism their religion.[22]

- Access to translators who are not also family and friends is best practice.[22]

- Women and girls may be reluctant to discuss delicate subjects in front of men, including male providers.[8,22]

- Understanding and recognizing religious and cultural values (*la familia, personalismo, respeto, espiritualidad,* and *coraje/valentía*) are essential to evaluation and treatment.[1–3,10,11,28]

- Collaboration with traditional healers may be necessary.[1,22]

- Safety, psychological first aid, and regulation skills must be established before implementing other evidence-based treatments.[1,22]
- Exposure work should never be done in the context of ongoing trauma.[1]
- The use of family stories, legends, *dichos* (proverbs), and *cuentos* (parables) is a valuable part of CM-TF-CBT[2,10,20,28,29] and other evidence-based therapeutic approaches such as Child-Centered Play Therapy.
- Focus on strength and resilience rather than vulnerability and disease.[6–8,11]
- Children and youth need to be engaged as partners in solving problems. Creating opportunities for young people to share their views and experiences is critical to their resilience.[6,11]

DISCLOSURE

The authors have nothing to disclose.

REFERENCES

1. Bryant B, Amaya-Jackson L. Children's narratives of forced migration: cultural factors, resilience, and treatment considerations for children at the border. J Am Acad Child Adolesc Psychiatr 2022;61(10S):S285.
2. De Arellano M, Danielson K, Felton J. In: Cohen J, Mannarino A, Deblinger E, editors. Children of Latino descent: culturally modified TF-CBT in trauma-focused CBT for children and adolescents: treatment Applications. Guilford Press; 2017. p. 253–79.
3. Flores L, Kaplan A. Addressing the mental health problems of border and immigrant youth. National Child Traumatic Stress Network; 2009. http://www.nctsn.org. Accessed January 9, 2022.
4. Fortuna L. Pros and cons: eliciting the trauma narrative during the asylum mental health evaluation. J Am Acad Child Adolesc Psychiatr 2020;59(10S):S3–4.
5. Fortuna L, Justine L, Lohr D, et al. Institute 1, systems of care and the needs of migrant youth: global and local responses. J Am Acad Child Adolesc Psychiatr 2022;61(10S):S123.
6. Lusk M, Sanchez G. Witness to forced migration: the paradox of resiliency. Hope Border Institute; 2021. https://hopeborder.org. Accessed January 10, 2022.
7. Lusk M, Terrazas S, Caro J, et al. Resilience, faith, and social supports among migrants and refugees from Central America and Mexico. J Spirituality Ment Health 2019;23(1):1–22.
8. Mujeres y niñas migrantes en Centroamérica se arriesgan en busca de un futuro mejor. blogs.worldbank.org. Published June 6, 2023. Accessed August 22, 2023. https://blogs.worldbank.org/es/latinamerica/mujeres-ninas-migrantes-buscan-futuro-mejor-centroamerica
9. Pierce K, Shapiro GL. Youth at the border: do no more harm. J Am Acad Child Adolesc Psychiatr 2020. https://doi.org/10.1016/j.jaac.2020.07.016.
10. Sanchez-Garcia G. In: Becerra C, Valdez G, Bustamante R, editors. Exploring resilience in migrant children from Central America and Mexico. YouTube; 2022.
11. Sanchez-Garcia G. Trauma and resilience among migrant children from Mexico and the northern Triangle Enroute to the United States. Open Access Theses & Dissertations 2022. Available at: https://scholarworks.utep.edu/open_etd/3627. Accessed August 22, 2023.

12. Cheatham A, Roy D. U.S. Detention of Child Migrants. Council on Foreign Relations. Published October 29, 2020. https://www.cfr.org/backgrounder/us-detention-child-migrants
13. Conradi L, Hendricks A, Merino C. V2 N3 2007 culture and trauma brief. The National Child Traumatic Stress Network; 2007.
14. De Vargas C. Clinical characteristics of migrant children living in shelters on the border. J Am Acad Child Adolesc Psychiatr 2022;61(10S):S286.
15. Estefan LF, Ports KA, Hipp T. Unaccompanied children migrating from Central America: public health implications for violence prevention and intervention. Current Trauma Reports 2017;3(2):97–103.
16. Murray LK, Cohen JA, Ellis BH, et al. Cognitive behavioral therapy for symptoms of trauma and traumatic grief in refugee youth. Child and Adolescent Psychiatric Clinics of North America 2008;17(3):585–604.
17. Stewart RW, Orengo-Aguayo R, Gilmore AK, et al. Addressing barriers to care among hispanic youth: telehealth delivery of trauma-focused cognitive behavioral therapy. Behav Ther 2017;40(3):112–8.
18. Valencia C, Fillingim RB, Bishop M, et al. Investigation of central pain processing in postoperative shoulder pain and disability. Clin J Pain 2014;30(9):775–86.
19. Gonzalez R, Ruiz A. Mi primer Libro de Dichos. Children's Book Press; 1995.
20. Ramirez J, Garcia T. 7 Tips to Engage in Mental Health Treatment: The Guatemalan Maya Families Living in the United States. National Hispanic and Latino Mental Health Technology Transfer Center Network. Published 2020. Accessed January 9, 2020. https://mhttcnetwork.org
21. Instituto Nacional de Estadísta, Geografia E Informática (INEGI) Religión. Censos y conteos. Población y Vivienda. Published January 1, 2010. https://www.inegi.org.mx/temas/religion/
22. Ramirez J, Garcia T. Cultural Aspects and Mental Health Disorders among Mexican American Children Youths, and Families. National Hispanic and Latino Mental Health Technology Transfer Center. Published July 10, 2020. Accessed January 9, 2022. https://mhttcnetwork.org
23. Cultura Maya. worldhistoryorg. Published online July 6, 2012. Accessed July 15, 2022. https://www.worldhistory.org/trans/es/1-11151/cultura-maya/
24. National Center on Cultural and Linguistic Responsiveness. Bridging Refugee Youth & Children's Services. https://brycs.org
25. Kibakaya EC, Oyeku SO. Cultural humility: a critical step in achieving health equity. Pediatrics 2022;149(2). https://doi.org/10.1542/peds.2021-052883. e2021052883.
26. Song S. Clinical considerations in working with unaccompanied minors in detention and community settings. J Am Acad Child Adolesc Psychiatr 2020; 59(10S):S3.
27. Stewart RW, Orengo-Aguayo R, Villalobos BT, et al. Implementation of an evidence-based psychotherapy for trauma-exposed children in a lower-middle income country: the use of trauma-focused cognitive behavioral therapy in El Salvador. J Child Adolesc Trauma 2020;14(3):433–41.
28. De Arellano MA. The national child traumatic stress Network: adapting trauma-focused treatments for diverse populations. The National Child Traumatic Stress Network; 2019. https://www.nctsn.org. Accessed January 9, 2022.
29. Echevarría Velez IS. Trauma-Focused Cognitive Behavioral Therapy: A Culturally-Modified Therapy to Work with Latino Children and Youths. National Hispanic and Latino Mental Health
30. National Hispanic and Latino Mental Health Technology Transfer Center (MHTTC) Network. mhttcnetwork.org. Accessed January 2022. https://mhttcnetwork.org

31. NCTSN learning center for child and adolescent trauma. NCTSN Learning Center; 2021. https://learn.nctsn.org.
32. Real Academia de la Lengua Española. Diccionario de la lengua española - Edición del Tricentenario. Published 2021. https://dle.rae.es.
33. Psychological First Aid Online. National Child Traumatic Stress Network. Accessed May 2023. https://learn.nctsn.org
34. Sellers JM. Folk wisdom of Mexico. Chronicle Books; 2005.
35. Shadid O, Sidhu SS. The mental health effects of migrant family separation. J Am Acad Child Adolesc Psychiatr 2021;60(9):1052–5.
36. Silliman D. Evangelicals Outgrow Catholics in Central America. ChristianityToday.com. Published February 13, 2023. Available at:https://www.christianitytoday.com/ct/2023/march/evangelicalism-grows-central-america-catholic.html. Accessed August 22, 2023.

Unaccompanied Children in the Office of Refugee Resettlement Care

Mawuena Agbonyitor, MD, MSc

KEYWORDS

- Unaccompanied children • United States border • Mental health • Trauma

KEY POINTS

- Unaccompanied children (UC) are children aged 17 years and younger who have no lawful immigration status in the United States and who do not have a parent or guardian in the United States available to provide care and physical custody.
- UC are cared for by the Office of Refugee Resettlement (ORR) under the Department of Health and Human Services.
- While under ORR care, the children receive a variety of services including case management for unification and health-care, legal, and education services.
- The Mental and Behavioral Health Services Team (MBHST) was created in 2019 and provides oversight and guidance around the mental and behavioral health of UC in ORR care. The MBHST is located within the Division of Health for Unaccompanied Children, which was created in 2017.

INTRODUCTION

The Office of Refugee Resettlement (ORR) is tasked with caring for unaccompanied children (UC) entering the United States. Following a referral from the Department of Homeland Security (DHS) or another federal entity, ORR is legally required to provide care to all UC from the time they enter ORR's custody until they are released to a vetted sponsor. Children are cared for in a variety of care provider programs across the country, including shelters, group homes, and foster care, among other types of settings. The goal is for children to ultimately be placed in care of a family member or qualified sponsor via a safe and timely release process. While in ORR care, ORR staff provide oversight around medical concerns that develop with the children and guide care providers in addressing children's mental health needs.

The Office of Refugee Resettlement

The Office of Refugee Resettlement falls under the supervision and guidance of the Administration of Children and Families, which is a division of the United States

Office of Refugee Resettlement, 330 C Street Southwest, Washington, DC 20201, USA
E-mail address: mawuena.agbonyitor@acf.hhs.gov

Child Adolesc Psychiatric Clin N Am 33 (2024) 141–149
https://doi.org/10.1016/j.chc.2023.09.001
1056-4993/24/Published by Elsevier Inc.

childpsych.theclinics.com

Department of Health and Human Services (HHS; **Fig. 1**). ORR has direct oversight of the UC Program and is tasked with ensuring all children in custody receive appropriate care and services. ORR funds care provider programs around the country, who provide direct care services to UC.

The Office of Refugee Resettlement was created in 1980 after the Refugee Act became law. Its mission is to provide people with critical resources needed to support their integration into American society. Oversight of services for UC was moved from the Immigration and Naturalization Service (INS) to ORR in 2002 when the Homeland Security Act created several changes to the federal government's immigration processes; this was formalized in 2003.[1]

Definition of Unaccompanied Children

UC are defined by 3 criteria (**Fig. 2**): (1) UC are children aged younger than 18 years, (2) are without lawful immigration status in the United States, and (3) have no parent or guardian in the United States, or no parent or legal guardian in the United States available to provide care and physical custody.[2]

UC are different from refugees; however, some UC can attain refugee status if they meet the appropriate criteria. Refugees are defined and protected by international law. The 1951 Refugee Convention[3] is a key legal document and defines a refugee as someone who "owing to well-founded fear of being persecuted for reasons of race, religion, nationality, membership of a particular social group, or political opinion, is outside the country of [their] nationality and is unable or, owing to such fear, is unwilling to avail [themselves] of the protection of that country; or who, not having a nationality and being outside the country of [their] former habitual residence, is unable or, owing to such fear, is unwilling to return to it."[3]

Additionally, UC are different from asylees, although UC may apply for asylum when entering or while within the United States. According to ORR "Asylees are individuals who, on their own, travel to the United States and subsequently apply for/receive a grant of asylum. Asylees do not enter the United States as refugees. They may enter as students, tourists, businesspersons, or even in undocumented status. Once in the U.S., or at a land border or port of entry, they apply to the Department of Homeland Security (DHS) for asylum. To qualify for asylum status, the person must meet the definition of a refugee and meet an application deadline. Asylum status permits the person to remain in the United States."[4]

Demographics of Unaccompanied Children in Office of Refugee Resettlement Custody

The number of UC referred to ORR care has increased substantially in the past decade, from 13,625 referrals in fiscal year 2012 to 128,904 referrals in fiscal year 2022 (October 2021–September 2022).[5] In fiscal year 2022, the majority of the children were male (64%) and teenagers—36% were aged 17 years, 36% were aged 15 to 16 years, and 13% were aged 13 to 14 years.[5] Most of the children in ORR custody came from countries in the Northern Triangle of Central America. In fiscal year 2022, 47% of children were from Guatemala, 29% were from Honduras, and 13% were from El Salvador (**Fig. 3**).[5]

UNACCOMPANIED CHILDREN PATHWAY INTO, THROUGH, AND OUT OF OFFICE OF REFUGEE RESETTLEMENT CARE
Unaccompanied Children Entry into Office of Refugee Resettlement Care

After apprehension by a federal agency, UC are transferred to ORR custody. Most children enter ORR care via the following pathway (**Fig. 4**): after crossing the border,

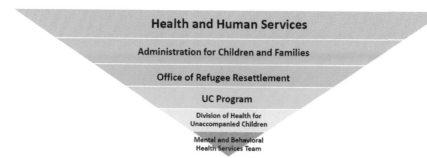

Fig. 1. Location of the Mental and Behavioral Health Services Team for the Unaccompanied Children Program within the U.S. Department of Health and Human Services.

children are taken into custody of Customs and Border Protection (CBP) under the Department of Homeland Security (DHS). Pursuant to the William Wilberforce Trafficking Victims Protection Reauthorization Act of 2008, barring exceptional circumstances, any department or agency of the Federal Government that has an unaccompanied child in custody is required to transfer the child to the Secretary of Health and Human Services (HHS) no later than 72 hours after determining that such child is unaccompanied. Within ORR care, many different factors enter in the consideration of the child's placement. Children are placed in the least restrictive placement that is appropriate to their needs. Placements range from shelters, to foster care or group homes (which may be therapeutic), staff secure or secure care facilities, residential treatment centers, or other special needs care facilities.[6] According to the ORR UC Program Policy Guide, "A secure care provider is a facility with a physically secure structure and staff able to control violent behavior. ORR uses a secure facility as the most restrictive placement option for an unaccompanied child who poses a danger to self or others or has been charged with having committed a criminal offense. A secure facility may be a licensed juvenile detention center or a highly structured therapeutic facility... A staff secure care provider is a facility that maintains stricter security

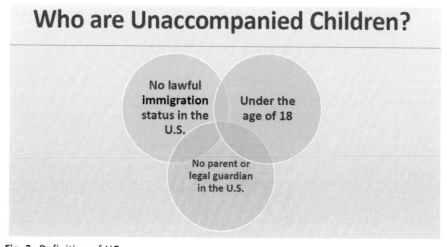

Fig. 2. Definition of UC.

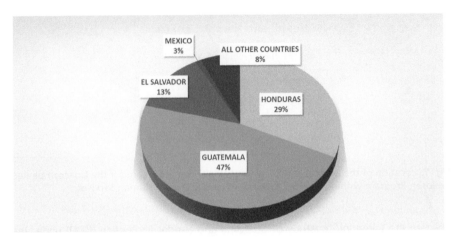

Fig. 3. Countries of origin of UC under ORR care in fiscal year 2022.

measures, such as higher staff to unaccompanied children ratio for supervision, than a shelter to control disruptive behavior and to prevent escape. A staff secure facility is for unaccompanied children who may require close supervision but do not need placement in a secure facility. Service provision is tailored to address an unaccompanied child's individual needs and to manage the behaviors that necessitated the child's placement into this more restrictive setting. The staff secure atmosphere reflects a more shelter, home-like setting rather than secure detention. Unlike many secure care providers, a staff secure care provider is not equipped internally with multiple locked pods or cell units."[7]

Of note, although most UC are referred to ORR care after being apprehended by immigration authorities while crossing the border, there are other situations that can lead to a child being placed directly in ORR custody. For example, there are special circumstances where children are referred to ORR by DHS when they are identified as unaccompanied in community settings, such as the airport. This was the case with the Afghanistan evacuation, where unaccompanied Afghan minors were taken into ORR custody at the airport under a preplanned unique procedure.

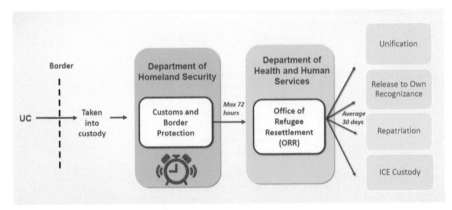

Fig. 4. UC pathway through federal custody.

Discharge from Office of Refugee Resettlement Care

A child may be discharged from ORR custody through several pathways. The most common method is via unification with a vetted qualified family member or nonrelative sponsor. During fiscal year 2022 127,447 UC were released to their sponsor, and the average length of stay in ORR care for a UC was 30 days.[5] Another discharge method includes release on one's own recognizance if the child turns 18 years of age while in ORR care. Similarly, a child may be released to US Immigration and Customs Enforcement custody if they turn 18 years old and cannot be released on their own recognizance, for example, if it is thought the child is of imminent danger to self or others. Finally, on the child or their legal guardian's request, at any age a child may be repatriated back to their home country.

Unification Process

The goal for UC in ORR care is unification with vetted sponsors via a safe, efficient, and timely process. Sponsors are adults and can include the child's parents, legal guardians, biological relatives, or individuals designated by the child's parents.

Unification procedures aim to ensure that vetted sponsors can provide for the physical and mental well-being of the child and to protect the child from smugglers, traffickers, or other individuals who may seek to victimize the child. Once a potential sponsor has been identified, they must complete a family reunification application. The reunification process also includes interviews, verification of the sponsor's identity and relationship to the child, background checks, home studies if indicated, and post-release planning.[6]

Once a child is released to a vetted sponsor, ORR's custodial responsibilities end. However, ORR has policies in place to promote the safety and well-being of UC by linking them to services after they have been released from ORR care and transition into a new community, as is required or permitted by statute.

HEALTH SERVICES GIVEN TO UNACCOMPANIED CHILDREN IN OFFICE OF REFUGEE RESETTLEMENT CUSTODY
General Health Services Provided to Unaccompanied Children

As noted above, children are placed in a variety of care settings while in ORR custody along a continuum of care. Children are placed in the least restrictive setting in their best interests. These settings include shelters, group homes (including those licensed as therapeutic), staff secure and secure placements, transitional foster care, long-term foster care, residential treatment centers, and influx care facilities (ICFs). ICFs are temporary facilities used during an influx (when the number of UC entering the United States exceeds ORR capacity) or emergency. They may be unlicensed or exempted from local licensing requirements; therefore, there are specified criteria that children must generally meet to be placed there, including lacking any known special needs (such as mental health or medical conditions).[6]

While in ORR care, children receive medical and mental health-care services, classroom education, social skills/recreation services, vocational training as appropriate, family unification services, access to legal support, and case management.

Shortly after placement, several assessments are conducted to identify needs to be addressed. If a youth reports a history of a mental health treatment when in CBP custody, children are transferred to ORR care with a medical summary form that contains the youth's historical diagnoses, medications (if indicated), and whether there is a need for further follow-up. Within 72 hours of admission, a case manager or mental health clinician performs a risk assessment that evaluates a child's need for appropriate support and supervision, especially if they have a history of being a victim or perpetrator of sexual abuse. This assessment is also done whenever a child transfers to another ORR placement. Within 5 calendar days of admission, the UC Assessment must be completed by a case manager or mental health clinician. This assessment collects information about the child's family structure, journey to the United States, medical history, educational history, legal history, and mental health (including substance use). It must be completed before release or transfer to another ORR placement. These assessments provide information with which a case manager will complete the child's Individual Service Plan that documents actions that have or will be implemented to address the child's reunification, legal, medical, and mental health needs.[6]

Within 2 business days of admission each child receives an initial medical examination (IME) by a medical professional.[6] The purposes of the IME are to assess general health, administer vaccinations in keeping with US standards, identify health conditions that require further attention, and detect communicable diseases, such as influenza and active tuberculosis. The IME is performed by a licensed health-care provider (medical doctor, doctor of osteopathy, nurse practitioner, or physician's assistant). The IME is based on a well-child examination, adapted for the UC population with consideration of screening recommendations from the American Academy of Pediatrics, the CDC, and the US Preventive Services Task Force. Children receive additional medical services while in ORR care depending on their needs—these include medical examinations for physical health concerns, routine medical and dental care, family planning services, emergency health services, prescribed medications and specialized diets, and mental health services.

Mental Health Care and Services for Unaccompanied Children in Office of Refugee Resettlement Care

All UC under ORR custody receive weekly individual therapy sessions provided by licensed or licensed-eligible mental health professionals referred to as "clinicians" who are most times also employees of the care placement where the child resides. When therapy is provided by a licensed-eligible clinician, it is under the supervision of a licensed clinician. Therapy sessions can consist of various therapeutic techniques, including psychoeducation, provision of coping strategies, brief supportive therapy, triage services, crisis intervention, and safety planning. The goals of individual counseling sessions are to monitor the child's progress with adaptation in the United States, assess postunification mental health needs, and evaluate and provide recommendations if acute mental health concerns develop. All UC also receive twice weekly, group counseling sessions that enhance the children's knowledge of supports and resources available to them and foster relationships with other children in the program. Finally, children receive family sessions with relatives in their home country and/or with their sponsor in the United States that provide the children opportunities to connect with family in a supportive environment and prepare the vetted sponsors and children for unification.

The above services are provided to all children, even those who have stable mental health, to encourage and promote resiliency. As shown in **Fig. 5**, the mental health of UC can fall anywhere along a health continuum. Although the majority of children in ORR care are considered to be in the "healthy to reacting" category ("reacting" implies some disruption in daily activities), some children may fall in the "injured to illness" category along this continuum. In these instances, such children are linked to other mental health services, including psychiatric evaluation and treatment from community providers, specialized therapy modalities from community therapists, intensive

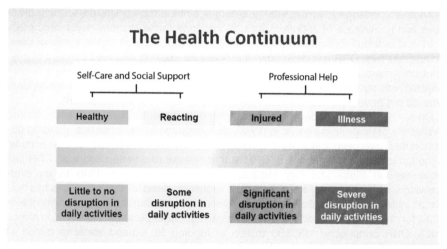

Fig. 5. Visualization of severity of mental health symptoms along the health continuum.

outpatient services within the community, substance use treatment from community providers, inpatient hospitalization in community child and adolescent psychiatric units, or treatment within residential treatment centers.

Oversight and guidance of the mental health of UC is provided by the Mental and Behavioral Health Services Team (MBHST) within the Division of Health for Unaccompanied Children (DHUC) in ORR. DHUC resides within the UC program (see **Fig. 1**). The MBHST was created in 2019 and currently consists of 2 child and adolescent psychiatrists, 2 licensed clinical social workers, 1 clinical advanced practice nurse specialist in child and adolescent mental health, and 1 clinical psychologist. The objective of the team is to oversee and monitor the mental and behavioral health of UC in ORR care, to provide guidance to other federal staff and care provider programs, to provide guidance to allied health-care professionals about ORR policies and systems, and to review and create mental and behavioral health-related policies and procedures.

There are some unique challenges to ensuring the provision of appropriate mental health care for UC in ORR custody. These include varied cultural beliefs about the origin and meaning of mental health symptoms and services, which can cause children to refuse services or treatment. Additionally, the transiency of symptoms due to adjusting to new circumstances and environments, or cultural differences in symptom presentation, can at times lead to misdiagnosis by psychiatric providers. Finally, as UC are, by definition, not residing with their parents or caregivers, it can be difficult to access collateral data on the child's social, developmental, and medical history.

There are also challenges within the ORR network of care that influence access to appropriate mental health care, which the MBHST is working to address. One is a need for a common goal and uniform approach to mental health care across the ORR network. At minimum, it is critical that children in ORR care are not harmed or traumatized and are provided with tools that will increase their resiliency or improve their health. To this end, MBHST is creating a unified mental health framework based on a trauma-informed approach that will be communicated to all levels of ORR and care program employees, from leadership to support staff. In this manner, an identical language and mission will be shared and applied among all those caring for UC who are in ORR custody.

Another challenge is proactively guarding against inappropriate prescribing practices and an overuse of antipsychotics, a challenge found in many psychiatric practices and settings throughout the United States, especially at higher levels of care. To address this, ORR has developed a process for seeking informed consent of psychotropic medications, which includes an external peer review component, where psychiatrists outside of ORR evaluate psychotropic medication regimens for children who do not have a parent, guardian, or sponsor that can provide consent.

Other challenges include limited availability of therapeutic placement beds, limited availability of postrelease services (PRS), and language/literacy barriers. Funding opportunities have been announced to address the shortage of therapeutic placements. Although custodial obligations of ORR end at release to a vetted sponsor, ORR has gone beyond these statutory requirements to offer voluntary PRS to an ever-growing segment of released UC and their sponsors. Need for these services has outpaced initial funding and staffing to provide services, causing limited availability of services for children and vetted sponsors to receive postreunification. However, in March 2023, ORR announced US$300 million in funding to expand services aimed at ensuring child safety and well-being, including PRS and other services for UC across the country. PRS includes timely referrals and connection to community resources, as well as intensive services in cases where additional support is necessary to address a child's specific needs or challenges. These referral and case management services are offered by a network of ORR-funded grantees across the United States. PRS can include help with school enrollment, support in finding and accessing physical health and mental health care, connections with local organizations, and other supports to ensure a child's well-being. Finally, there are language and literacy barriers—within care programs, English and Spanish language staff are readily available; however, interpreters must often be used for children speaking other languages or dialects. When searching for mental health services in the community, it can be quite challenging finding providers who can accommodate non-English languages, including Spanish. ORR reminds providers that it is their duty to render care to patients no matter the language used and that interpreters should be requested when needed.

SUMMARY

Before entry into the United States, the experiences of UC place them at risk for mental health problems. The Office of Refugee Resettlement's UC Program seeks to provide children with mental health support across a health continuum beginning at the time they enter ORR's custody until discharge to a suitable sponsor. Challenges exist with accessing culturally appropriate and timely pediatric mental health services while under ORR care, and after they are released to their vetted sponsors. ORR, DHUC, and the MBHST are working to mitigate these challenges to ensure that children receive the mental health care they need in ways that are meaningful to them.

CLINICS CARE POINTS

- Within 2 business days of admission, each child receives an IME by a medical professional.
- Within 72 hours of admission, a case manager or mental health clinician performs an Assessment for Risk that evaluates the child's need for appropriate support and supervision.
- Within 5 calendar days of admission, the UC Assessment must be completed by a case manager or mental health clinician. This assessment collects information around the child's

family structure, journey to the United States, medical history, educational history, legal history, and mental health.

- All UC under ORR custody receive weekly individual and group therapy sessions provided by licensed or licensed-eligible mental health professionals referred to as "clinicians."
- More intensive care is available through community providers, treatment programs and psychiatric hospitals.
- Children also receive family sessions with relatives in home country and/or with their sponsors in the United States through any appropriate form of communication (ie, over the phone, video chat, or in person if possible).

REFERENCES

1. About the Program Office of Refugee Resettlement and Office of the Administration for Children and Families. (2022, September 2). Available at: https://www.acf.hhs.gov/orr/programs/ucs/about.
2. Office of Refugee Resettlement. (2021, March 17). Unaccompanied Children Program Information. Available at: https://www.acf.hhs.gov/orr/unaccompanied-children-info.
3. Convention and Protocol Relating to the Status of Refugees. (2023, March 20). Retrieved from UNHCR USA web site: Available at: https://www.unhcr.org/3b66c2aa10.html.
4. Office of Refugee Resettlement. (2023, August 9). Fact Sheet Subject: Eligibility for ORR Benefits and Services – Asylees. Available at: https://www.acf.hhs.gov/sites/default/files/documents/orr/orr_fact_sheet_asylee.pdf.
5. Unaccompanied Children Facts Sheet and Data. (2023, February 24). Retrieved from Office of Refugee Resettlement An Office of the Administration for Children and Families: Available at: https://www.acf.hhs.gov/orr/about/ucs/facts-and-data.
6. ORR Unaccompanied Children Program Policy Guide. (2023, March 21). Retrieved from Office of Refugee Resettlement An Office of the Administration for Children & Families: Available at: https://www.acf.hhs.gov/orr/policy-guidance/unaccompanied-children-program-policy-guide.
7. Office of Refugee Resettlement. (2023, August 2). ORR Unaccompanied Children Program Policy Guide: Guide to Terms. Available at: https://www.acf.hhs.gov/orr/policy-guidance/unaccompanied-children-program-policy-guide-guide-terms.

Understanding the Legal Rights and Mental Health Needs of Unaccompanied Immigrant Children in US Government Custody and Beyond

Leecia Welch, JD

KEYWORDS

- Unaccompanied children • Trauma • Mental health • Office of Refugee Resettlement
- Immigrant rights • *Flores* Settlement Agreement

KEY POINTS

- Unaccompanied children have mental health rights rooted in the *Flores* Agreement, the US Constitution, federal statutes, and international law.
- The Office of Refugee Resettlement (ORR) has made efforts to address unaccompanied children's mental health needs, but additional policy changes, resources, and workforce investments are needed.
- Clinicians can play an important role in supporting the mental health needs of children through collaboration with the *Flores* team, other legal advocates, and ORR to create a more fully operational trauma-informed immigration system that respects the mental health rights of children.

INTRODUCTION

Over the past 7 years, I have interviewed hundreds of unaccompanied children in my role as counsel on the *Flores v. Garland* case. I have met children in the Donna, Texas border facility, unlicensed influx facilities, and emergency intake sites (EISs) at military bases, former mining barracks, and convention centers. I have spoken with children at all levels of the Office of Refugee Resettlement (ORR) network of licensed providers and contractors, including numerous shelters, residential treatment centers (RTCs), juvenile detention centers, and hospital psychiatric units. Each of these children has their own story, but common themes across the population include (1) tremendous bravery in the face of extremely challenging life circumstances, (2) hope for a new life free from abuse, human rights atrocities, and fear of death, and (3) desire for opportunities to succeed, thrive, and feel the love of their families.

Children's Rights, 88 Pine Street, Suite 800, New York, NY 10005, USA
E-mail address: lwelch@childrensrights.org

Child Adolesc Psychiatric Clin N Am 33 (2024) 151–161
https://doi.org/10.1016/j.chc.2023.10.007
1056-4993/24/© 2023 Elsevier Inc. All rights reserved.

These interviews have repeatedly demonstrated to me that the US immigration system was not designed to address the trauma unaccompanied children have experienced and, frequently, this system is causing them harm. Unaccompanied children have mental health rights established by the *Flores* Settlement Agreement, the US Constitution, federal statutes, and international law. For many years, the US government has been aware of the ways in which our immigration system exacerbates children's trauma, and although the Biden administration has made some improvements, there is significant work to be done to develop a system that is trauma-informed and responsive to the mental health needs of the thousands of children who come to our country each year seeking safe harbor.

Clinicians can play an important role in supporting the mental health needs of children both while they are in immigration custody and once they are released to families. In collaboration with the *Flores* team, other legal advocates, and ORR, clinicians can help create a safer, more trauma-informed immigration system, as well as help mitigate the impact of the harms experienced by children on an individual level.

OVERVIEW OF TRAUMA THAT UNACCOMPANIED CHILDREN MAY EXPERIENCE

In the past 10 years, more than 600,000 immigrant children have come to the United States and entered federal immigration custody.[1] Currently, most of these children are from Honduras, Guatemala, and El Salvador, and cross into the United States through the southern border.[1]

Children arriving at the US border without a parent or legal guardian are categorized as "unaccompanied children."[2] Even when children arrive at the US border with family members, such as grandparents, aunts, uncles, or adult siblings, they may be categorized as "unaccompanied" and separated from their adult caregiver (who is transferred to Immigration and Customs Enforcement custody).[3–5] Unaccompanied children are initially detained by the US Customs and Border Protection (CBP) agency, a division of the Department of Homeland Security.[6] Within 72 hours, these children must be transferred to the custody of ORR, which is the division of the US Department of Health and Human Services (HHS) responsible for their care.[2,7] Most of these children have family living in the United States with whom they hope to reunite or join, but those who do not may remain in ORR custody for prolonged periods of time.[8(p6),9]

Each of these children has a unique journey, but the majority have experienced a great deal of physical and mental trauma, including while they were still in their home countries, as they made their journeys to the United States, and while crossing the border.[4,10–12] Traumas experienced in their home countries include war, genocide, forced displacement, gang and drug cartel violence, lack of food and basic necessities, and abuse and death of a caregiver or family member.[4,10,11] In addition, many children travel hundreds of miles and cross multiple international borders by foot, bus, or atop freight trains. During their journey, unaccompanied children often experience additional traumatic events, such as physical and sexual violence, human trafficking, separation from family and other caregivers, and hazardous and unsafe travel and living conditions.[4,10(pp4–5),11]

Once children cross the US border, they remain at risk of having traumatic experiences. In CBP custody, for instance, they may face stress-inducing conditions, including freezing temperatures (the facilities have been referred to as "la hielera"—meaning "icebox"), lack of adequate food and water, sleep deprivation, unsanitary conditions, separation from adult family members and siblings, and abusive treatment by border patrol officers.[4(pp13,15,26,44),13,14] CBP facilities are often described by youth as cinder block or soft-sided tent jails with unsafe and inedible food, with only mats and mylar blankets for sleeping, no natural light, limited access to showers, and no opportunity to contact family members.[4(p15)] Since July 2022, CBP conditions have improved, but the most recent *Flores* monitoring report noted ongoing concerns relating to the separation of children from parents, lack of sleeping mats, lack of food for young children, lack of showers, and inadequate medical services.[13] Despite generally lacking child welfare training or experience with trauma-informed practices, CBP officers are responsible for screening children for signs of trafficking and determining whether they are unaccompanied.[10(pp4–5),15,16] These screenings have the potential to be traumatic as children are often asked to recount the harms they experienced in their home country and on the journey, without the support of family members.

Once they have been screened, CBP then transfers unaccompanied children to the custody of ORR, which is responsible for "promptly" placing the child "in the least restrictive setting that is in the best interests of the child."[4] ORR contracts with a network of about 300 providers in 27 states to provide unaccompanied children with shelter, case management, basic educational services, recreation, counseling, and medical services.[17,18] ORR is required to promptly release unaccompanied children to appropriate sponsors (usually family members who agree to take custody and provide care), and care providers must assign case managers to children to facilitate their safe and timely release.[18(p18),19] Unaccompanied children spend an average of one month in ORR custody; however, children who have greater mental health needs and are placed in RTCs or secure settings tend to have much longer lengths of stay — some spending many months or even years waiting to be released to a sponsor.[1,4,9,20(p9)] For example, an analysis of data of children's length of stay from November 2017 to March 2020 showed that children who spent time in an RTC had an average length of stay of 236.3 days, children who spent time in a therapeutic staff secure facility had an average length of stay of 246.3 days, and children who spent time in an out-of-network RTC had an average length of stay of 327.2 days.[20(p9)] According to the most recent data available from ORR, the average length of stay in ORR care for children overall has been reduced from 102 days in 2020 to 27 days in 2022.[1,21] More recent data are not available regarding the average length of stay for children who spent time in an RTC or other therapeutic setting.

The ORR provider network has a wide variety of placement types, sizes, and levels of restrictiveness, including foster homes, small and large congregate care placements, secure and staff-secure facilities (juvenile detention-type settings), and RTCs.[4,12,15] A significant number of unaccompanied children live in large-scale shelters with secured perimeters that house hundreds of children at a time.[4] The size of ORR's shelters range from a 1400-bed former Walmart Supercenter to group homes that serve less than 10 children.[22] Regardless of size, children spend their days in the facility, are not permitted to attend schools in the community, and do not enjoy the liberties typically afforded to young people in the United States.[17] Children and investigators have reported that the educational services and recreational activities at ORR facilities are inadequate.[9(pp22–23),23(pp20–23)] Children in ORR facilities may also experience stressors related to language barriers and lack of cultural competence, prolonged separation from family and restricted communications, lack of information about the status of their release to sponsors, lack of individualized mental health support, lack of appropriate policies and practices concerning administration of psychotropic medications, and conditioning release to family on mental health stability.[4,9,24–26] During my own interviews of children who had prolonged stays in ORR custody, they have consistently reported feeling isolated, overly regimented, and hopeless.[4,26–28]

As of March 31, 2023, only about 13% of children in ORR custody lived in community-based foster homes or smaller group homes where children attend local public school and enjoy a greater sense of normalcy.[29] ORR has been criticized for continuing to build up a network of large-scale, highly restrictive congregate settings instead of community-based foster homes.[9,30,31(pp52)]

OVERVIEW OF THE MENTAL HEALTH RIGHTS OF UNACCOMPANIED CHILDREN
Flores Settlement Agreement

In the 1980s, unaccompanied children from Central America increasingly fled to the United States to escape violence and hardships caused by civil wars. One of those children was named Jenny Flores. When Jenny made her way to the United States from El Salvador to be reunited with her mother, she was instead detained by the Immigration and Naturalization Service (INS) (the precursor agency to CBP) in a 1950s-style hotel surrounded by chicken wire on top and all around the perimeter.[32,33] Jenny was detained in a room with unrelated men, women, and children, and she spent her days confined to the hotel grounds with nothing to do.[32,33] There was no school, reading materials, or activities for the children and no standards whatsoever for their care.[32,33] Jenny had a cousin in the United States with legal status, but the INS refused to release children to anyone who was not a parent or legal guardian.[32,33] Jenny's mother did not have legal status, and if she had presented herself to the INS to get her daughter, she likely would have been deported to a war-torn country where her husband had been killed.[32,33]

In 1985, a group of lawyers, which I would later join, filed a case called *Flores v. Meese* (who was the US Attorney General at that time) on behalf of Jenny and a class of similarly situated children in federal immigration custody.[32] After more than a decade of litigation, the case was finally settled in 1997 by the Clinton Administration.[18] The *Flores* Settlement set national standards for the "detention, release, and treatment" of immigrant children in the custody of the US government.[18(p9)] Before the Settlement no such standards existed.

Broadly speaking, the *Flores* Settlement requires:

- Safe and humane treatment of children in the immediate aftermath of apprehension;
- Prompt placement of children in licensed dependent care facilities; and
- Release to parents, relatives, and other reputable sponsors without unnecessary delay.

The *Flores* Settlement was designed to ensure that vulnerable immigrant children receive the same child welfare protections as other children in government custody in foster care systems across the country. With limited exceptions, unaccompanied children must be placed in licensed facilities that "comply with all applicable state child welfare laws and regulations."[18] They also must be held "in the least restrictive setting" appropriate based on their age and needs.[18] The *Flores* Settlement also entitles unaccompanied children to:

- "Appropriate mental health interventions";
- An individualized needs assessment and plan;
- One individual counseling session with trained social work staff per week; and
- Two group counseling sessions per week.[18]

The *Flores* Settlement remains an enforceable consent decree under the court supervision of US District Judge Dolly Gee in the Central District of California. Therefore, the *Flores* legal team continues to represent all children in federal immigration custody and has the authority to interview children wherever they are being detained, to tour facilities, and to obtain monthly data about the children in custody.[18] Over the years, the *Flores* legal team has filed multiple motions to enforce the Settlement when the government has violated its terms, including motions focused on addressing the mental health needs of unaccompanied children.

In 2018, for example, the *Flores* legal team brought a motion to enforce the Settlement when our team was alerted to the fact that children in ORR custody were in RTCs without justification (ie, a licensed psychologist or psychiatrist had not determined they posed "a risk of harm to self or others") and were being administered psychotropic medications without staff first obtaining a court order or getting informed consent from a person authorized to provide consent, which violates Texas law. The lack of an informed consent process was particularly problematic because it was coupled with a lack of oversight over potentially harmful prescribing practices. Judge Gee ruled that the government had "breached . . . the *Flores* Agreement in the course of administering psychotropic medications."[24] She ordered that children should only go to restrictive RTCs when they posed a danger to themselves or others and that ORR must follow Texas child welfare laws and regulations governing psychotropic medications.[24]

In 2021, the *Flores* legal team filed a motion to enforce the Settlement focused on the Biden administration's ongoing reliance on EISs in the aftermath of the backup at the border and extreme overcrowding at the Donna CBP facility.[34,35] We highlighted the fact that conditions at some EISs were so harmful that children were experiencing acute mental health symptoms, including panic attacks, self-harm, and suicidal ideation.[4,34,36] At Fort Bliss EIS, for example, we observed children packed into soft-sided tents—some housing as many as 900 children—and forced to sleep doubled up on bunk cots.[4,34] The boys' tent had a strong stench likely due to failure to clean clothes and linens often enough; youth complained of not being able to shower for over a week, no recreation, no education, and feeling like prisoners.[4,34]

These conditions significantly impacted children's mental health.[37] One youth detained at Fort Bliss shared: "I felt anguished and hopeless . . . you spend the day in bed, surrounded by thousands of kids, with thousands of thoughts racing through your head."[4,34] Another youth shared: "Because I've been here so long, I've been getting a lot of anxiety, and my blood pressure has gone up. I used to be able to cope with my anxiety and breathe through it, but now I feel like I've given up. I feel like I'll never get out of here."[4] Pursuant to a settlement reached after our team filed the motion to enforce, the previously standard-less EISs now must operate in accordance with influx facility standards and protocols are in place in the event emergency operations are ever used again.[38]

Trafficking Victims Protection Reauthorization Act of 2008

Another important source of legal protection for unaccompanied children is the William Wilberforce Trafficking Victims Protection Reauthorization Act of 2008 (TVPRA). The TVPRA strengthened federal trafficking laws and created a variety of procedural rights for unaccompanied minors.[39] For the first time, Congress set standards for the treatment of children in federal immigration custody, addressed the provision of mental health services, and adopted child welfare principles, including the "best interests of the child" standard.[40]

The TVPRA established that children from noncontiguous countries (such as El Salvador, Guatemala, and Honduras) must be referred to ORR for screening and placement in the "least restrictive setting" within 72 hours and then released to a family member or placed in a foster home or ORR shelter pending their removal hearing—all of which reinforces entitlements originating from the *Flores* Settlement.[39] The TVPRA also created new entitlements to legal advocacy, including the right to a legal orientation presentation (called a "Know Your Rights" training); the right "to the greatest extent practicable" to have access to legal "counsel to represent them in legal proceedings or matters and protect them from mistreatment, exploitation, and trafficking"; and the opportunity to have a child advocate, when eligible, to promote the best interest of the child.[39] Under the TVPRA, children from contiguous countries (Mexico and Canada) are entitled to a screening for signs of trafficking, a determination of whether they have a "credible fear of returning to their home country," and a determination of whether they can make an independent decision to voluntarily depart before being turned around at the border.[39] Further, the TVPRA eliminated the one-year asylum filing deadline for unaccompanied children, modified the asylum process for children to make it less adversarial, and expanded Special Immigrant Juvenile Status protections.[41]

In addition, the TVPRA gave the Secretary of HHS the responsibility for determining when a home study must be conducted before the release of a child in ORR custody to a sponsor.[40] Under current ORR guidance, home studies are generally required before release for children who experienced "a severe form of trafficking," have been "a victim of physical or sexual abuse under circumstances that indicate the child's health or welfare has been significantly harmed or threatened," have a disability, or whose sponsor "clearly presents a risk of abuse, maltreatment, exploitation or trafficking to the child based on all available objective evidence."[40] Children for whom home studies are conducted are also entitled to post-release services, which are designed to connect children and their sponsors to community resources.[40]

US Constitution and Statutes

Unaccompanied children also have rights under the US Constitution, including protections pursuant to the Due Process Clause of the Fifth Amendment, the Freedom of Association Clause of the First Amendment, and the Due Process and Equal Protection Clauses of the Fourteenth Amendment.[20(pp19–36),42] For example, the Fifth Amendment states "no person . . . shall be compelled in any criminal case to be a witness against himself, nor be deprived of life, liberty or property without due process of law."[43] Similarly, the Fourteenth Amendment bars states from denying "any person the equal protection of the laws."[44]

In the children's immigration context, detained unaccompanied minors have due process rights to freedom "from unnecessary physical restraint and confinement for medical treatment, and to familial association."[20,45] In practice, this means that when the government detains children in its custody, they are entitled to various procedural protections to reduce the risk of erroneous deprivation of liberty, including notice of the reason they are being placed in restrictive settings and hearings to contest prolonged placement in restrictive settings.[46]

Unaccompanied minors are also entitled to the protections of a wide range of federal statutes including Title VI of the Civil Rights Act of 1964, which establishes the right to be free from discrimination based on race, color, religion, sex, or national origin,[42,47] and Section 504 of the Rehabilitation Act. Section 504 is particularly important in supporting the mental health needs of unaccompanied minors because it protects children with disabilities from discrimination and requires equal access to all benefits and services in federal programs or state programs receiving federal funding.[48] Under Section 504, "disability" is defined as having "a physical or mental impairment which substantially limits one or more major life activities."[48,49]

International Human Rights

Unaccompanied minors also have rights under international law, most importantly, protections found in the United Nations (UN) Convention on the Rights of the Child (CRC).[10(p6)] The United States remains the only UN country that has signed but not ratified the CRC, demonstrating that although the United States supports the intent behind the CRC, it is unwilling to be held legally accountable. Legal experts believe that ratification of the CRC would establish the US government's "obligation and accountability to address the holistic needs and rights of all children—including providing the highest quality of education, health and disability services; protection from exploitation, violence, family separation and bias in the juvenile justice system."[50] Nevertheless, the CRC provides an important framework for ensuring unaccompanied children receive the fundamental freedoms and conditions that they deserve, including respecting that the "best interests of the child" should be a primary consideration in all decision-making, the right to health, the right to due process, and the right to be free from all forms of violence.[10(p6)]

Addressing the Mental Health Needs of Unaccompanied Children

As highlighted above, unaccompanied children in government custody are entitled to a wide range of legal protections to support their mental health, including rights under the *Flores* Settlement, the TVPRA, the Due Process Clause, Section 504, and international law.

Like many systems, ORR providers face mental health workforce challenges, and the lack of intensive mental health services in shelters can result in children being transferred to more restrictive RTCs and hospital settings.[12,15] In recent years, ORR has taken some steps to address these challenges, including partnering with the National Center for Traumatic Stress Network to develop trainings on trauma as it pertains to unaccompanied children and providing greater access to an array of treatment options.[12(pp33–34),15(pp48–56)] Clinicians interested in partnering with ORR providers could play a vital role in filling gaps in ORR's continuum of mental health services.[4]

Greater attention must also be paid to the mental health needs of unaccompanied children as they are released to sponsors. A recent report on the mental health needs of unaccompanied minors by the American Academy of Pediatrics and Migration Policy Institute highlights promising community-based practices from across the country that clinicians could consider expanding into their own communities.[8(p6)] The report also provides a roadmap for ways in which interested clinicians can support the mental health needs of unaccompanied children, including by participating in multidisciplinary coalitions, assisting with trainings in community settings, and volunteering at welcome centers or community-based clinics.[8(pp35–36)]

SUMMARY

Unaccompanied children often face tremendous trauma and adversity before, during, and after their journeys to the United States. There is growing awareness of the impact of these traumas; there are promising trauma-based interventions to address them; and unaccompanied children have legal rights to mental health services under the *Flores* Agreement, the Constitution, and international and federal laws. Although lawyers for unaccompanied children continue to advocate for a more trauma-informed immigration system, including greater access to these services, clinicians can simultaneously provide crucial immediate support to children while they are in government custody and as they transition to living with their families in US communities.[4]

ACKNOWLEDGMENT

Special thanks to Anna Hackel for her helpful comments, edits, and citation formatting assistance on this article.

REFERENCES

1. U.S. Dept. *Of health and human services (HHS), administration of children and families (ACF), Office of refugee resettlement (ORR)*, 2023, Fact sheets and data, Available at: https://www.acf.hhs.gov/orr/about/ucs/facts-and-data. Accessed October 2, 2023.
2. Homeland Security Act of 2002, 6 U.S.C. § 279(g) (unaccompanied children ('UCs") are children who arrive at the border who: (A) have no lawful immigration status in the United States; (B) have not attained 18 years of age; and (C) with respect to whom—(i) there is no parent or legal guardian in the United States; or (ii) no parent or legal guardian in the United States is available to provide care and physical custody.).
3. Bryant E., Children are still being separated from their families at the border, 2022, Vera Institute of Justice, Available at: https://www.vera.org/news/children-are-still-being-separated-from-their-families-at-the-border. Accessed October 2, 2023.
4. Matlow R., Desai N., Adamson M., et al., Guidance for mental health professionals serving unaccompanied children released from government custody, 2021, Stanford Early Life Stress and Resilience Program, National Center for Youth Law, Center for Trauma Recover and Juvenile Justice, Available at: https://youthlaw.org/sites/default/files/attachments/2022-03/2021_Guidance-for-Mental-Health-Professionals-Serving-Unaccompanied-Children-Released-from-Government-Custody.pdf. Accessed October 2, 2023.
5. TRAC Immigration. Growing numbers of children try to enter the U.S., 2022. Available at: https://trac.syr.edu/immigration/reports/687/. Accessed October 2, 2023.
6. Kandel W.A., Unaccompanied alien children: an overview, 2021, Congressional Research Service, Available at: https://sgp.fas.org/crs/homesec/R43599.pdf. Accessed October 2, 2023.
7. Trafficking Victims Protection Reauthorization Act (TVPRA) of 2008, 8 U.S.C. § 1232(b).
8. Beier J. and Fredricks K., A path to meeting the medical and mental health needs of unaccompanied children in U.S. communities, 2023, American Academy of Pediatrics, Migration Policy Institute, Available at: https://www.migrationpolicy.org/sites/default/files/publications/aap-mpi_unaccompanied-children-report-2023_final.pdf. Accessed October 2, 2023.
9. Desai N., Adamson M., Cohen L., et al., Child welfare & unaccompanied children in federal immigration custody: a data and research based guide for federal policy makers, 2019, National Center for Youth Law, Stanford University Dept. of Emergency Medicine, Available at: https://youthlaw.org/sites/default/files/attachments/2022-02/Briefing-Child-Welfare-Unaccompanied-Children-in-Federal-Immigration-Custody-A-Data-Research-Based-Guide-for-Federal-Policy-Makers.pdf. Accessed October 2, 2023.
10. Ataiants J, Cohen C, Riley AH, et al. Unaccompanied children at the United States border, a human rights crisis that can be addressed with policy change. J Immigr Minor Health 2018;20(4):1000–10. Notably, the Committee on the Rights of the Child, which is the body that interprets the CRC, has specifically published a General Comment on the "Treatment of unaccompanied and separated

children." This comment notes that States should "take into account the fact that unaccompanied children have undergone separation from family members and have also, to varying degrees, experienced loss, trauma, disruption and violence. The profound trauma experienced by many affected children calls for special sensitivity and attention in their care and rehabilitation.".

11. Corona Maioli S, Bhabha J, Wickramage K, et al. International migration of unaccompanied minors: trends, health risks, and legal protection. Lancet Child & Adolescent Health 2021;5(12):882–95.

12. U.S. Dept. of Health and Human Services (HHS), Office of Inspector General. Care provider facilities described challenges addressing mental health needs of children in HHS custody. 2019. Available at: https://oig.hhs.gov/oei/reports/oei-09-18-00431.pdf. Accessed October 2, 2023.

13. Notice of Filing of Juvenile Care Monitor Rep. by Dr. Paul H. Wise, Flores v. Reno, No. 85-4544 (C.D. Cal. Sept. 15, 2023), ECF No. 1360.

14. Op. from 9th Cir. Ct. App., Flores v. Reno, No. 85-4544 (C.D. Cal. Aug. 15, 2019), ECF No. 624.

15. U.S. Dept. of Health and Human Services (HHS), Office of Inspector General. The Office of Refugee Resettlement needs to improve its oversight related to the placement and transfer of unaccompanied children. 2023. Available at: https://oig.hhs.gov/oas/reports/region6/62007002.pdf. Accessed October 2, 2023.

16. KIND. The impact of the asylum ban on children seeking safety in the United States. May 2023. Available at: https://supportkind.org/wp-content/uploads/2023/05/23_The-Impact-of-the-Asylum-Ban-on-Children-Seeking-Safety-in-the-United-States.pdf. Accessed October 2, 2023.

17. U.S. Dept. of Health and Human Services (HHS), Administration of Children and Families (ACF), Office of Refugee Resettlement (ORR). ORR influx care facilities for unaccompanied children. Updated May 26, 2023. Available at: https://www.acf.hhs.gov/sites/default/files/documents/orr/icf-uc-fact-sheet.pdf.   Accessed October 2, 2023.

18. Stipulated Settlement Agreement, Flores v. Reno, No. 85-4544 (C.D. Cal. Jan. 17, 1997) (children traveling with parents or guardians are processed by the U.S. Immigration Customs and Enforcement ("ICE") agency. ICE has discretion to release or detain families. Under the Obama and Trump administrations, families were being held in family detention centers for extended periods.) (despite the intention and spirit of these requirements, as noted above, ORR house a significant number of children in large-scale shelter facilities that are akin to orphanages. The size, restrictiveness and isolated nature of these facilities continues to be a serious problem.).

19. Trafficking Victims Protection Reauthorization Act (TVPRA) of 2008, 8 U.S.C. § 1232(c)(2).

20. Order re Cross-Mots. for Summ. Judgement at 21, Lucas R. v. Becerra, No. 18-5741, 2022 WL 2177454 (C.D. Cal. Mar. 11, 2022), ECF No. 376.

21. U.S. Dept. of Health and Human Services (HHS), Administration of Children and Families (ACF), Office of Refugee Resettlement (ORR). Fact sheet: unaccompanied children (UC) program, 2023. Available at: https://www.hhs.gov/sites/default/files/uac-program-fact-sheet.pdf. Accessed October 2, 2023.

22. Barker K. and Kulish N., Inquiry into migrant shelters poses dilemma: what happens to the children?, 2019, New York Times, Available at: https://www.nytimes.com/2019/01/05/us/southwest-key-migrant-shelters.html. Accessed October 2, 2023.

23. Mathews K., Logsdon L., Lew P., et al., The detention of immigrant children with disabilities in California: a snapshot, 2019, Disability Rights California, Available at: https://www.ndrn.org/wp-content/uploads/2020/03/Detention_of_Immigrant_Children.pdf. Accessed October 2, 2023.
24. Order re Pls.' Mot. to Enforce Class Action Settlement, Flores v. Reno, No. 85-4544 (C.D. Cal. July 30, 2018), ECF No. 470.
25. Decl. of Leecia Welch in Supp. of Pls.' Resp. to Juvenile Coordinator's Interim Reports, Flores v. Reno, No. 85-4544 (C.D. Cal. Nov. 23, 2020), ECF No. 1039-8.
26. Wood LCN. Impact of punitive immigration policies, parent-child separation and child detention on the mental health and development of children. BMJ Paediatr Open 2018;2(1):e000338.
27. Song SJ. Mental health of unaccompanied children: effects of U.S. immigration policies. BJPsych Open 2021;7(6):e200.
28. Alvarez K. and Alegria M., Understanding and addressing the needs of unaccompanied immigrant minors: depression, conduct problems and PTSD among unaccompanied immigrant minors, 2016, American Psychological Association, Available at: https://www.apa.org/pi/families/resources/newsletter/2016/06/immigrant-minors. Accessed October 2, 2023.
29. U.S. Dept. of Health and Human Services (HHS), Administration of Children and Families (ACF), Office of Refugee Resettlement (ORR). Bed capacity report January to March 2023.
30. Pls.' Resp. to ORR Juvenile Coordinator's June 4, 2021 Interim Report, Flores v. Reno, No. 85-4544 (C.D. Cal. June 21, 2021), ECF No. 1136.
31. Nagda J., Reimagining children's immigration proceedings: a roadmap for an entirely new system centered around children, 2020, Young Center for Immigrant Children's Rights, Available at: https://static1.squarespace.com/static/597ab5f3bebafb0a625aaf45/t/5f9acdcb38fc5b520e882eb1/1603980749320/Reimagining+Children%E2%80%99s+Immigration+Proceedings_Young+Center+for+Immigrant+Children%27s+Rights.pdf. Accessed October 2, 2023.
32. Compl., Flores v. Reno, No. 85-4544 (C.D. Cal. July 11, 1985), ECF No. 1.
33. Interview with Carlos Holguin, 2018, National Public Radio, Available at: https://www.npr.org/2018/06/22/622678753/the-history-of-the-flores-settlement-and-its-effects-on-immigration. Accessed October 2, 2023.
34. Mem. in Supp. of Mot. to Enforce Settlement re Emergency Intake Sites, Flores v. Reno, No. 85-4544 (C.D. Cal. Aug., 9, 2021), ECF No. 1161-1.
35. U.S. Dept. of Health and Human Services (HHS), Office of Inspector General. Operational challenges within ORR and the ORR emergency intake site at Fort Bliss hindered case management for children, 2022. Available at: https://www.oig.hhs.gov/oei/reports/OEI-07-21-00251.pdf. Accessed October 2, 2023.
36. Desai N., de Gramont D. and Miller A., Unregulated & unsafe: the use of emergency intake sites to detain immigrant children, 2022, National Center for Youth Law, Available at: https://youthlaw.org/sites/default/files/attachments/2022-06/EIS%20Briefing%20FINAL.pdf. Accessed October 2, 2023.
37. Montoya-Galvez C., Migrant children endure "despair and isolation" inside tent city in the Texas desert, 2021, CBS News, Available at: https://www.cbsnews.com/news/immigration-migrant-children-fort-bliss-tent-city-texas/. Accessed October 2, 2023.
38. Stipulated Settlement of Pls.' Mot. to Enforce Settlement re Emergency Intake Sites, Flores v. Reno, No. 85-4544 (C.D. Cal. June 22, 2022), ECF No. 1256-1.
39. Mathur R. and Cervantes W., Legal protections for unaccompanied minors in the trafficking victims Act of 2008, 2014, First Focus Center for the Children of

Immigrants, Available at: https://firstfocus.org/wp-content/uploads/2014/08/Legal-Protections-for-Unaccompanied-Minors-in-the-Trafficking-Victims-Protection-Act-of-2008.pdf. Accessed October 2, 2023.

40. Rodriguez J., Protections for unaccompanied children in the trafficking victims protection reauthorization Act of 2008 (TVPRA), In: *Where we stand: a 20-year retrospective of the unaccompanied children's program in the United States,* 2022, U.S. Committee for Refugees and Immigrants (USCRI), The Children's Village, Available at: https://refugees.org/wp-content/uploads/2022/09/Chapter-Three-Protections-for-Unaccompanied-Children-in-the-Trafficking-Victims-Protection-Reauthorization-Act-of-2008-TVPRA.pdf. Accessed October 2, 2023.

41. KIND. What are the TVPRA procedural protections for unaccompanied children?, 2019. Available at: https://supportkind.org/wp-content/uploads/2019/04/KIND-TVPRA-talking-points-4.1.19-FINAL.pdf. Accessed October 2, 2023.

42. Title VI of the Civil Rights Act of 1964, 42 U.S.C. § 2000d.

43. U.S. CONST. amend. V.

44. U.S. CONST. amend. XIV.

45. Order Granting Pls.' Mot. for Classwide Prelim. Inj., Ms. L. v. U.S. Immigration and Customs Enforcement, 302 F. Supp. 3d 1149 (S.D. Cal. June 26, 2018) (No. 18-0428), ECF No. 83.

46. National Center for Youth Law., *Practice advisory: preliminary injunction in* Lucas R. v. Becerra, 2022, Available at: https://youthlaw.org/sites/default/files/attachments/2022-10/22%2010%2031%20Practice%20Advisory.pdf. Accessed October 2, 2023.

47. American Bar Association. Rights of immigrants: questions and answers. 2022. Available at: https://www.americanbar.org/groups/crsj/projects-and-initiatives/civil-rights-civics-institute/rightsofimmigrants/. Accessed October 2, 2023.

48. Order re Defs.' Mot. to Dismiss and Pls.' Mot. for Class Certification, Lucas R. v. Becerra, No. 18-5741, 2022 WL 2177454 (C.D. Cal. Nov. 2, 2018), ECF No. 126.

49. U.S. Dept. of Health and Human Services (HHS), *Fact sheet: your rights under Section 504 of the rehabilitation act,* 2006, Available at: https://www.hhs.gov/sites/default/files/ocr/civilrights/resources/factsheets/504.pdf. Accessed October 2, 2023.

50. Lichtsinn H, Goldhagen J. Why the USA should ratify the UN convention on the rights of the child. BMJ Paediatr Open 2023;7(1):1–7.

Advocacy and Policy
A Focus on Migrant Youth

Abishek Bala, MD, MPH[a],*, Jessica Pierce, MD, MSc[b],
Karen Pierce, MD, DFAACAP, DLFAPA[c], Suzan Song, MD, MPH, PhD[d]

KEYWORDS

• Advocacy • Policy • Migrant • Refugee • Mental health • Asylum

KEY POINTS

- A comprehensive approach is essential to effectively advocate for the mental health of migrant children, considering their unique migration experiences and circumstances.
- To promote policies and champion the cause of migrant children's mental health, it is vital to comprehend the complex interplay among biopsychosocial factors, social determinants of health, and the larger social frameworks that influence their well-being.
- Achieving meaningful change for this vulnerable population requires interdisciplinary collaboration and a collective effort to dismantle systemic barriers and enhance their access to mental health care.

VIGNETTE: ADVOCACY CULTIVATES ADVOCACY

Picture a clinical encounter in which you meet a migrant child who lacks English proficiency and displays signs of psychological distress. How can you conduct an evidence-based, unbiased assessment and create a tailored plan without making generic assumptions? In such a scenario, perhaps your standard practice is to use an interpreter to ensure informed consent and accurate communication. Perhaps you turn to reliable and culturally validated instruments like the Strengths and Difficulties Questionnaire or Child Behavior Checklist to enhance the assessment process and mitigate implicit bias in the qualitative interview.[1] The fact that providers like you recognize the need for interpreters for preferred-language access and culturally competent tools for screening in this context—and likely consider them to be "obvious" standards of care—underscores the power of advocacy. Clinic policies, funding for interventions like interpreters, and education on best practices often derive from the actions of advocates and community partners working together to effect

[a] Central Michigan University, 1000 Houghton Avenue, Saginaw, MI 48602, USA; [b] University of Michigan, 1500 East Medical Center Drive, Ann Arbor, MI 48109-5277, USA; [c] Northwestern University Department of Psychiatry, 2634 N Dayton ST, Chicago, Il 60614, USA; [d] Boston Children's Hospital, 1 Brookline Place, Suite 552, Boston, MA 02445, USA
* Corresponding author.
E-mail address: bala1a@cmich.edu

Child Adolesc Psychiatric Clin N Am 33 (2024) 163–180
https://doi.org/10.1016/j.chc.2023.09.004
1056-4993/24/© 2023 Elsevier Inc. All rights reserved.

childpsych.theclinics.com

change at the organizational and legislative levels. What's more, as the provider treating this patient, you may identify another area of concern or inequity that deserves exploration to improve care. Advocacy cultivates advocacy.

INTRODUCTION

Child and adolescent psychiatrists devote their clinical and research efforts to improving the mental health and well-being of children, delivering care, and advancing innovation across diverse practice settings. Wherever their professional homebase, child psychiatrists can embrace an additional role, that of physician advocate, to lend their voices and devote their time to support causes and policies that promote the health of the patients and populations they serve or work to reform policies that harm them.[2] Although there are myriad issues that physician advocates can take up in support of children affected by mental illness, a helpful point for effecting meaningful change is to consider the social determinants of mental health and examine how physicians might work to combat the inequities and adverse consequences of the societal and political status quos.[3,4]

Migrant children and families are particularly vulnerable to social inequality in many forms—income, education, employment, food and housing security, social exclusion and discrimination, structural violence, and health care access and affordability—such that it has been suggested that immigrant status itself may serve as an important social determinant of health.[5,6] Indeed, extensive literature details the mental health concerns, psychosocial stressors, and treatment challenges facing migrant youth, as well as the successful interventions, beneficial policies, and encouraging resilience and strength exhibited by these young people across the globe.[7–9] For the 36 million international migrant children, the stakes are unquestionably high for their mental health and well-being, whereas the cards of social justice may feel insurmountably stacked against them.[10] Child psychiatrists are uniquely positioned to effect direct and personal change for migrant families through individual patient care; to learn from and support migrant families through community engagement; and to highlight the inequities and promote successful reforms at the policy level.

UNDERSTANDING ADVOCACY

Advocacy efforts can feel daunting to individual practitioners due to the gravity of the causes they undertake to address and the sheer size of the systems they aim to modify. A helpful means of conceptualizing advocacy as an accomplishable endeavor is to break it down into three levels of engagement: individual or patient-level advocacy; community or organization-level advocacy; and population-level or legislative advocacy.[11] Later, we outline specific opportunities for child psychiatrists to advocate in each of these arenas on behalf of migrant children.

Practicing advocacy at any of these intervention levels, physicians should begin by educating themselves on the facts and varied perspectives of an issue. Proceeding with a surface-level understanding of a complex subject can be ineffective at best and harmful at worst. Recognizing one's own knowledge limitations and especially one's own cultural perspectives and the importance of seeking and incorporating the perspectives of others, physician advocates work best when collaborating across settings and with varied individuals or groups who are dedicated to—or directly affected by—the cause. Communication is an imperative skill to use in practicing advocacy, but it is important to note that this "communication skill" encompasses not only the ability to relay one's expertise or persuade an audience on the merits of an argument but also the capacity to *listen* to every viewpoint and to interpret the nonverbal cues of others involved in the issue.[11–14] From the first moment of self-education to the ultimate act of intervention, practicing advocacy requires humility and a persistence that is rooted in social conscience, rather than self-aggrandizement.

Of note, the American Medical Association (AMA) expressed clearly in their Declaration of Professional Responsibility (2001) that they view medicine to hold a "social contract with humanity," citing an imperative to combat the injustices that affront the health and well-being of humankind. The document specifically identifies advocacy as an obligation of the physician, with a mandate to advance "social, economic, educational, and political changes that ameliorate suffering and contribute to human well-being."[15] Physicians must pursue this work through a lens of professionalism and ethics, ensuring that the basic tenets of beneficence and nonmaleficence are maintained while supporting the autonomy and justice of the individual patients and populations served.[11,15,16]

POLICY AND POPULATION HEALTH

Individual patients and communities are impacted significantly by policies and laws implemented at the local, state, and federal levels. For physician advocates aiming to effect change on a population scale, a crucial first step is to ensure that they understand the forms of government in the regions and countries in which they practice, as well as the key entry points for citizens and advocacy groups to interface with lawmakers there.[17] Exploring governmental Web sites and the online advocacy centers of professional organizations such as the AMA, the American Psychiatric Association (APA), the American Academy of Pediatrics (AAP), and the American Academy of Child and Adolescent Psychiatry (AACAP) can be a helpful starting point for digesting the structures and procedures of governmental bodies. Visiting similar online resources pertaining to other nations may be helpful guides for physician advocates outside the United States, in addition to the World Health Organization (WHO) and the various United Nations (UN) bodies pertaining to the populations or specific causes at hand.

Domestic and international policies related to migrant health are complicated and efforts to support or reform them can be divisive and contentious for the societies and individuals involved. Extensive literature and educational materials already exist delineating the specifics of policies relating to migrant health in the United States and abroad; offering a comprehensive policy review here is beyond the scope of this article and would surely do injustice to the depth and nuance required to adequately encapsulate the issues.[18,19] Instead, we examine broad policy concerns and feature a concrete legislative advocacy effort pertaining to migrant children's mental health, highlighting for child psychiatrists "where and how" they might intervene as advocates at the population level. For in-depth inquiry, we direct readers to the specific governmental entities interacting with migrants in the legal sphere—the US Department of State, Immigration and Customs Enforcement, US Citizen and Immigration Services, the Department of Homeland Security, Office of Refugee Resettlement (ORR), and relevant state legislatures—and to the independent and nonpartisan organizations such as the Council on Foreign Relations (CFR.org) and the Migration Policy Institute (migrationpolicy.org) for further information.

As an important primer, Article 24 of the UN Convention on the Rights of the Child recognizes the right of every child to the highest attainable standard of health and the obligation of state parties to ensure for them the provision of necessary medical care and health care services.[20] This article includes the protection of the rights of all children *without discrimination*, irrespective of their migration status. Despite this treaty, several countries continue to maintain policies that limit access to health care for migrant populations.[21] Also of note, the United States is the only member nation not to have ratified the treaty; although the United States has expressed clear reasons for this and it remains a controversial position politically and among the public, the decision has carried broad implications for the health and well-being of migrant children and the domestic and international policies that affect them.[22]

Recognizing immigration status as a social determinant of health, immigration law naturally affects health and health policy for migrants.[5,6,23] Policy affects resource availability and shapes health behaviors through incentives and deterrents, thereby shaping overall health care systems and outcomes for individuals and populations. Simply put, anti-immigration policies may directly affect health care access and outcomes for migrant children and families.[23–25] A 2021 Kaiser Family Foundation study found that among the US non-elderly population, a significant proportion of lawfully present immigrants (25%) and undocumented immigrants (46%) lacked health insurance, in contrast to only 8% of citizens. Moreover, noncitizen children were more prone to being uninsured compared with their citizen peers. Citizen peers were less likely to have insurance if one of their parents was a noncitizen.[26] As legal barriers interfere with the ability to obtain insurance, individuals may avoid care altogether. The costs associated with seeking health care and the cultural stigma surrounding mental health specifically may deter individuals from seeking services; this may explain why migrant children are likely to have reduced utilization of health care services, including mental health care.[27] Recognizing these policy-related inequities, advocacy efforts might support integrated care models offering services such as health care, case management, and immigration consultation in a "one-stop-shop" effort to increase resource affordability, accessibility, and quality for migrant families.[28]

In unprecedented times like the COVID-19 pandemic, vulnerable populations face myriad barriers that interfere with health care access and delivery. For example, as highlighted by Hill and colleagues and the National Immigration Law Center, COVID relief bills like the CARES Act for economic relief and health care options for the COVID-19 pandemic required documents showing an immigration status that allows for a work permit as well as a Social Security Number to qualify.[23,29] These restrictions excluded many families and children from receiving assistance during a tumultuous time and further contributed to feelings of alienation and distrust.[30,31] In addition to limiting health care access, the government invoked Title 42 U.S.C. section 265 of the 1944 Public Health and Service Act to suspend the right to seek asylum, citing concerns surrounding the spread of COVID-19.[32] These actions, including family separation and expulsion, have had direct and detrimental impacts on the mental health of the migrants involved.[33–36] As a result of this policy, migrants already in the country were likely to avoid seeking health care, including testing and treatment of COVID-19 due to fears of deportation.[23] Policies that govern resource accessibility and shape health care behaviors among migrants widen health disparities and exacerbate the burden of mental illness.

HOW CAN CHILD AND ADOLESCENT PSYCHIATRISTS ADVOCATE FOR MIGRANT CHILDREN AND FAMILIES?
Individual-Level Advocacy

Individual-level advocacy carries an asterisk when the individual in question is a minor, as children are dependent on—and thrive within—the family unit. This is no less true for children living apart from their families, as in the case of unaccompanied minors or children engaged in the child welfare system. To practice individual-level advocacy in the pediatric population is to consider each element of the child's functional circle:

the child; the caregivers (immediate and extended family, foster family, group homes, and so forth); and the child's local supports (school, neighborhood, religious community, and so forth).[37] In this section, we reflect on opportunities for child psychiatrists to engage in individual-level advocacy on behalf of migrant children and their families, considering the unique circumstances and operative challenges inherent to the work (**Table 1**).

Clinical Care as Advocacy

Direct patient care can be conceptualized as a form of advocacy, as it promotes the health and well-being of the patient. Advocacy opportunities within clinical care become especially apparent for child psychiatrists when they consider the holistic presentation of the patient and examine the social determinants of mental health relevant to the situation.[4] An important first step in this sort of advocacy is for providers to reflect on their own potential cultural biases and preconceptions, recognizing that stereotyping and prejudice, however subtle or unconscious, can result in misdiagnosis and unequal treatment.[7,38,39] In this way, child psychiatrists can practice advocacy by

Table 1	
Individual-level advocacy efforts	
Relationship levels	**Opportunities for Engagement**
Direct Clinical Care	• Cultural humility and bias recognition among providers • Institutional accountability for equitable care • Language equity: • In-person interpreters vs language line • Translation for written patient education materials • Insurance/payor limitations: • Prior authorizations • Out-of-network exceptions or appeals • Financial aid for specific therapies • Refer for urgent subspecialty medical examinations • Parent/caregiver mental health care • Family therapy referrals • Unaccompanied or child welfare-involved youth: • Reliable sources for collateral information • Identify legal decision-maker(s) • Access to health coverage
Beyond the Office	• Contextual factors (eg, food/housing insecurity, utilities access, transportation, childcare, unemployment): • Compile written resource guides (translated) • Write letters of support • Complete health assessments for government aid • Partner with social workers, case managers • School interventions: • Write letter for 504 Plan or IEP • Request language interpretation (child and family) • Trauma-informed interventions for behavior • Peer concerns: acculturation, bullying, stigma
Nontreatment Relationship	• Forensic asylum evaluations • Become trained (medical, psychological, both) • Partner with academic institution or local legal aid group to reach clients • Write a medicolegal report • Testify in court (if asked)

approaching their own patient care within a framework of cultural humility and institutional accountability and encouraging the same for their practice colleagues or trainees in the academic setting.[40] Broadening this lens beyond the individual assessment and treatment plan, psychiatrists can work as advocates in helping their patients navigate complex health care systems, contend with insurance and payor barriers, and access equitable care across disciplines.[41]

Dobson and colleagues put forward a helpful framework for considering the actions of individual-level advocates in the context of providing clinical care, outlining a distinction between what they have termed clinical agency and paraclinical agency. Providers engage in clinical agency when they work to overcome a barrier to an individual patient's immediate medical needs within the clinic setting.[12] For child psychiatrists working with migrant children and families, this may include actions such as securing patient education materials in the child's preferred language, pursuing insurance authorization for a non-covered medication, seeking financial assistance for a specialized treatment not covered by public funding or solely available "out of network" for private insurances, or arranging for an urgent subspecialty medical examination to address possible comorbid conditions affecting the psychiatric presentation.[12,41] Recognizing the important role of caregiver stress and the possibility that migrant parents may have endured significant traumatic experiences themselves, child psychiatrists might enact clinical agency by placing referrals for the parent's own mental health care, parent management training, or family therapy, acknowledging that such measures may improve outcomes for the child.[42–44] Finally, for unaccompanied children or those otherwise engaged in the child welfare system, practicing clinical agency may involve obtaining reliable collateral information from foster families, extended relatives, or care workers who know the child well before solidifying diagnoses and ensuring that the appropriate legal decision-maker is identified before enacting treatment plans.[45] The nuances of custody for unaccompanied minors and their sponsors working with the ORR can be confusing and questions about access to health care coverage and community resources may arise in real time in the clinic setting.[28] Partnering with social work and external case managers or community agencies who are supporting the child may assist in advocating for comprehensive mental health care for these youth.

It is worth noting that the efforts described here as clinical agency-related advocacy work could simply be conceptualized as basic elements of practicing pediatric psychiatry requisite for providing the standard of care. Indeed, Dobson and colleagues comment that most physicians involved in their study identified clinical agency tasks as "an integral part of their role" and an obligation for "all practicing physicians," questioning whether to consider it advocacy at all.[12] Importantly, however, child psychiatrists may believe that they lack the agency to engage in these elements of clinical care in certain practice settings due to infrastructure problems, health systems limitations, time constraints, or payor demands and insufficient reimbursement. In addition, literature consistently suggests that standards of care often go unmet for minoritized and marginalized groups, as social disadvantage and structural discrimination hinder both the access to and quality of health care services.[39,46] National health care quality data suggest that black patients experience lower quality on 60% of health care measures compared with white patients and low-income patients experience lower quality on 62% of health care measures compared with high-income patients, citing access to care, provider bias, and insurance accessibility as clear contributors. For example, breast cancer screening rates differ significantly between uninsured and insured patients (38.5% vs 79.9%); tobacco-use screening and smoking cessation rates are lower among Latinos compared with non-Latino whites; and Medicare Advantage enrolled black patients show lower rates of control for hypertension, blood sugar management, and cholesterol than non-Latino whites.[46] For migrant families, barriers to the standard of care can be profound, relating to language and communication, health literacy and cultural conceptions of illness, knowledge about payor systems and one's legal rights to information and services, and outright fear that engaging with the medical system may carry legal repercussions or threaten immigration status.[47] Although these hurdles certainly require broader advocacy efforts to surmount (discussed further below), the clinical agency of an individual provider who invests extra time and effort to overcome these challenges in the service of delivering the standard of care—even to one vulnerable patient in one clinical interaction—is an instrumental act of advocacy.

Advocacy Beyond the Office

Outside the examination room, child psychiatrists engage in *paraclinical agency* when they work to overcome barriers related to social determinants of health that affect patients in their daily environment.[3,12] Advocacy efforts might relate to mitigating contextual stressors such as food insecurity, housing instability, utilities access, transportation challenges, childcare needs, and family financial strain or unemployment.[44] Partnering with social workers, case managers, legal advocates, and local charities or nonprofits, child psychiatrists can compile resource guides (translated into preferred languages, when possible) that detail local food banks, housing supports, employment training opportunities, and financial aid programs.[4] Advocating for a specific patient by writing a letter attesting to the adverse effects of a given contextual factor on the patient's physical and mental well-being (eg, "Dear Landlord...Overcrowding and the presence of mold in the apartment have precipitated asthma exacerbations and worsened anticipatory panic attacks...Any help you can offer in eliminating these environmental strains to support [patient's] health and well-being would be most appreciated...") has been shown to prompt positive change.[48] Advocates might complete health assessments for paperwork relating to governmental social services or write letters in support of non-emergent transportation for patients to attend medical and therapy appointments.[49,50] Engaging the expertise of social work and case management colleagues can be vital in these paraclinical agency efforts for families.

Schools represent another clear target for paraclinical agency at the individual patient level. In line with the standard of care for outpatient practice, child psychiatrists should advocate for appropriate school accommodations for their patients, writing letters in support of 504 Plans or Individualized Education Plans (IEPs) when indicated.[51] With the family's permission, child psychiatrists can take a step further in advocating for specific school-based interventions relating to the migrant child's unique needs, such as language interpretation (for child and caregivers), acculturation-related adjustments as students adapt to unfamiliar educational systems, trauma-informed approaches to behavioral concerns, and general awareness of stigma-related issues with peers.[44,52] Schools may also offer resources for the contextual factors affecting mental health, particularly with respect to food insecurity and before/after school care options, having access to federal programs and funding.[53,54]

Nontreatment-Related Individual Advocacy

Beyond the direct doctor–patient relationship, child psychiatrists can practice individual-level advocacy by volunteering their time to conduct psychological evaluations and write medicolegal reports for children and/or caregivers who are applying for asylum. In this context, physicians evaluate and document the objective physical and/

or psychological sequelae of torture or ill treatment, comment on the consistency be-tween the client's reported history and the clinical findings, and formulate a profes-sional opinion regarding possible medical or psychological risks of return to the country of origin.[55–57] Typically, this is done outside the therapeutic context (ie, for a single assessment without an anticipated ongoing treatment relationship) and in collaboration with stakeholders in the legal sphere.[40] Clinical evaluations can be highly impactful for asylum seekers—one study demonstrated that 89% of cases with an accompanying medical evaluation were granted asylum, compared with the national average of 37.5% without one (data from 2000 to 2004).[58] To our knowledge, data have not been collected specifically for child asylum cases with accompanying med-ical or psychological affidavits, but we suspect the inclusion of a medicolegal docu-ment positively supports the application.

Although there is no formal certification or governing body to license psychiatrists in conducting forensic asylum evaluations, a network of nongovernmental organizations working in partnership with multiple academic medical centers across the country pro-vides training for interested physicians following a set of international standards known as the Istanbul Protocol, established by the UN Office of the High Commis-sioner for Human Rights; these collaborations can be found in Ferdowsian and col-leagues and via the organization Physicians for Human Rights (PHR.org).[55,56,59] There are no formalized standards specific to conducting asylum evaluations in the pediatric population, but Ferrera and Giri provide helpful guidance on issues unique to assessing child asylum seekers. Interviewing a child in this context requires that close attention be paid to the psychological effects of recounting the story and the risks of re-traumatization. This is particularly pertinent when children have been sepa-rated from their most trusted adults, as they may lack a clear supportive figure to turn to in the duress of the process. In addition, questions may arise regarding whether children (especially unaccompanied minors) can give informed consent to undergo these evaluations at all and how to safeguard the privacy of their story once it has been documented.[57] Ultimately, if child psychiatrists are interested in this work, we advise that they seek guidance from the established collaboratives and experts active in the field, to ensure that their well-meaning advocacy efforts uphold the ethical mandate to first do no harm, both psychologically and legally.

COMMUNITY-LEVEL ADVOCACY

Physicians have the expertise and social capital to effect meaningful change on behalf of vulnerable groups in the form of community-level advocacy, promoting health and well-being in their local and regional spheres.[11] Interestingly, many of the efforts described above as individual-level advocacy can be broadened beyond the individ-ual patient to reach communities overall.[40] In this section, we conceptualize community-level advocacy in four sectors: schools and school boards; community centers, charities, and nonprofit organizations; healthcare systems and insurance/payors; and local media and press (**Table 2**).

Schools and School Boards

Working with schools and school boards is an important and generally accessible point of entry for engaging in community-level advocacy. Although writing a letter requesting accommodations for a single student may be crucial for that individual, it could have scalable impact if extrapolated to the school at large. It is common for im-migrants and refugees to settle in residential and neighborhood clusters; thus, if a psy-chiatrist treats a patient who is attending a particular school, it is likely that other

Table 2
Community-level advocacy efforts

Community-level Advocacy Efforts	
Schools and School Boards	• Educational presentations for teachers/administrators: • Mental health of migrant youth • Trauma-informed care • Resilience models • Stigma and bullying • Acculturation, inclusivity, identify formation • School-based mental health care services (funding for): • Mental health literacy programs • Anti-bullying measures • Trained therapists in trauma-focused modalities • Peer support programs • Language equity: • In-person interpreters vs language lines • Translation for written information for parents
Community Centers, Charities, and Nonprofit Organizations	• Contextual factors (eg, food/housing insecurity, utilities access, transportation, childcare, unemployment): • Network with local agencies • Become a referral center for clients to services • Speak on a panel or at an education session • Support funding efforts • Volunteer time • Develop institutional coalitions or partnerships: • Health and legal aid clinics • Special populations clinics • Health systems/neighborhood coalitions • Peer support programs
Health Systems and Insurance/Payors	• Barriers to care: • Access to treatment (geographic, transportation) • Parity in coverage for medical vs mental health care • Interpreter and translation services • Equitable care: • Cultural sensitivity training for crisis support teams • Education on migrant health for emergency departments • Create specialized clinics supported by health system funding
Local Media and Press	• Writing: • Essays and opinion editorials • Books • Blogs • Social media posts • Give interviews: • Written articles • Television or documentary film • Radio • Podcasts • In-person media events

migrant children are also enrolled.[44] Child psychiatrists can give educational presentations to teachers and administrators or contribute to panel discussions on pertinent issues like trauma-informed care and resilience models, mental health stigma and bullying, and the importance of culturally inclusive activities and supports for students contending with acculturation and identity formation concerns.[9,44,60–63] In this way, child psychiatrists practice education as advocacy, extending their clinically developed skills as content experts and communicators into their role as child advocates.[11]

School boards represent another step toward scalability, as child psychiatrists can advocate for system-level changes. Beyond accommodating for academic and emotional needs and implementing mental health literacy and anti-bullying measures, schools are increasingly being viewed as important sites for delivering mental health care.[64] Child psychiatrists can petition school boards and local legislatures to develop, fund, and grow in-school mental health services. Specifically, delivering trauma-focused cognitive behavioral therapy (CBT) or Narrative Exposure Therapy via trained professionals in educational settings can promote positive outcomes for migrant youth who have experienced trauma and are contending with the stressors of resettlement.[60] For youth coping with mental health concerns outside the context of trauma—bereavement, anxiety, adjustment, or other conditions—supportive therapy and general CBT delivered through schools would also be beneficial.

Community Centers, Charities, and Nonprofit Organizations

Given their "on the ground" location and integration with the populations they serve, community centers, local charities, and nonprofit organizations provide natural collaboration partners for physicians.[11] The contextual factors relating to social determinants of health are addressed most accessibly by engaging with existing and embedded community supports. Here, the needs of the parent or family unit may be more pressing areas for advocacy intervention than those of the child individually, with efforts focused on mitigating problems of financial strain, unemployment, and caregiver support. Advocacy partners might include housing nonprofits and shelters, legal aid organizations, or language and job-training charities.[44] Peer support programs have shown progress in improving social connectedness and mental well-being among migrant adults, as participants respond well to mentors with shared experiences.[64] For adolescents struggling with identity formation in the context of acculturation, peer programs may be instrumental. Engaging with community organizations staffed by and serving individuals and families of similar backgrounds and with relatable experiences may offer important supports, cultivating trust and resilience.[9,64] Child psychiatrists can practice advocacy by educating themselves about local agencies and community programming, networking with those actors, and learning from and supporting their efforts.[65]

Health Care Systems and Insurance/Payors

Within health care systems, physicians can practice organizational advocacy by working to eliminate barriers to care, inequity in assessment and treatment planning, and payor limitations on coverage and access to services. Li and Franklin outline a helpful plan of approach for enacting organizational advocacy, adapting John P Kotter's eight stages of change to the psychiatric health care setting. They advise starting by conveying a sense of urgency about the need for change, creating and communicating a vision for how the change might take shape, recognizing and consolidating victories in the enactment of change, and solidifying effective approaches for ongoing success.[66,67] Following this model, advocacy projects might include: establishing or improving interpreter and translation services for in-person and written psychoeducation efforts; implementing cultural sensitivity training for local crisis intervention teams or emergency departments; or creating specialized clinics within a health care system to treat unaccompanied minors.[9,44] Whatever the chosen area for intervention, advocates should understand that organizational change takes time and often requires nuance and attention to political and hierarchical undertones within the system; realistic goal setting and solution-focused proposals carry the greatest potential for success.[67]

Local Media and Press

Child psychiatrists can practice community-level advocacy by engaging with the media, literally lending a voice to the cause. The narrative nature of psychiatry is a feature that draws many physicians to the field, recognizing the power of story and the impact of personal plot developments on the individual psyche. Child psychiatrists can adapt their expertise as elicitors of stories (ie, clinical interviewers) and their skills as narrative writers (eg, years of documenting psychodynamic formulations or biopsychosocial assessments) to convey to the lay public the personal side of mental health care and the advocacy needs therein. Storytelling can humanize technical science and complex health care policies, motivating the audience to engage in the issues.[68–70]

Media advocacy may take many forms, including writing personal essays or opinion editorials for local (or even national) publications, engaging with the public or press on social media platforms, or giving interviews over the radio, on television, on podcasts, or at public media events; Barron and colleagues provide a detailed "how-to" guide for psychiatrists interested in enacting media advocacy in each of these forms.[71] As psychiatrists take up the pen, they should be mindful of the fact that they are not the owners of the stories they tell, but rather the safekeepers of other people's stories, entrusted with the privilege and responsibility of relaying them. Even de-identified, a patient's personal narrative remains personal, and writers have an obligation to avoid sensationalizing or embellishing, even in the service of effecting meaningful change. In addition, writers should keep tabs on their own perspectives and roles in the stories they tell, remaining watchful for the insidiously seductive savior complex and the ethical quandaries inherent in balancing objectivity with compassion, especially in politically charged subject matters like immigrant and refugee policy.[72]

POLICY-LEVEL ADVOCACY

Political lobbying, grassroots campaigning, and legislative efforts represent fundamental components within the realm of advocacy.[17] Advocacy through policy development typically begins with professionals engaging policy makers to emphasize the significance of a problem and its potential societal impact. According to the WHOs Advocacy for Mental Health Package, the initial step involves gathering objective evidence to demonstrate the problem's severity. Policy makers consider various factors, such as public opinion, financial implications, and power dynamics when weighing the risks and benefits of a policy decision. The subsequent step is policy implementation, which involves aligning public interests with the political interests of legislators. Success in advocating for a policy proposal should then be framed within the larger political landscape, highlighting the investment and desired outcomes (**Table 3**). Strengthening alliances between advocates and policy makers can further enhance the campaign's success.[17,73] For instance, the New York Times' exposé in 2023 on migrant child labor exploitation sparked a significant public outcry and a demand for change.[74] By shedding light on the harsh conditions and resulting fatalities affecting these children, the case was made for protecting their rights and improving their bio-psychosocial outcomes. The approach was both informative and persuasive, prompting a bipartisan response and compelling the government to take immediate action.[75]

One prominent example of a mental health advocacy nonprofit organization that engages in legislative advocacy and readily partners with psychiatrists is the National

Table 3
Policy-level advocacy efforts

Policy-level Advocacy Efforts	
Advocacy Forms	• Support grassroots efforts • Lobby local councils and legislatures • Lobby state legislatures • Lobby federal legislatures • Local or national media engagement
Steps in Legislative Advocacy (WHO 2005)	• Identify problem and express its severity • Objective evidence (scientific research) • Public opinion • Outline policy goals and execution plan • Financial implications • Power dynamics and politics • Risks vs benefits • Implement policy • Align public and political interests • Anticipate hurdles • Measure outcomes • Objective data • Qualitative/narrative data • Financial impact • Public opinion
Helpful Partners	• Grassroots political campaigns • Nonprofit organizations • Local, state, or national advocacy groups • For example, NAMI, SCAN • Professional organizations • For example, AMA, AAP, APA, AACAP • Current or past legislatures or political figure heads • Members of the press, celebrities, artists, athletes

Alliance on Mental Illness (NAMI) in the United States. NAMI provides support, education, and advocacy for individuals and families affected by mental health conditions. NAMI lists its "Policy Priorities" online and regularly lends its support to bills and policy proposals that would benefit the mental health of migrant children (NAMI.org). Another notable example is the political advocacy arm of the nonprofit Save the Children, known as Save the Children Action Network (SCAN). SCAN actively promotes mental health issues by bridging government relations with grassroots activism to engage policymakers across the United States (savethechildrenactionnetwork.org). Like NAMI, SCAN partners with physician advocate to elevate individual voices and effect change. While just two examples among many, these organizations highlight the practice of working collaboratively with various stakeholders to define government responsibilities, allocate resources, and integrate mental health into broader health care systems.[73] The advocacy and government affairs committees within physician professional organizations such as the APA, AAP, AACAP, and AMA provide additional resources and partners for collaboration, addressing individual and population mental health concerns in addition to issues pertaining to the practice and profession of psychiatry.

The marriage between advocacy and policy is exemplified by the "Mental Health in International Development and Humanitarian Settings Act" or MINDS Act (S. 767 and H.R. 1570), a bipartisan bill codeveloped and supported by more than 20 organizations (including SCAN, AAP, and UNICEF USA) in response to the significant mental health impact of disasters, trauma, and poverty on children globally. The bill addresses mental health and psychosocial support in foreign assistance, aiming to promote best practices, establish a global mental health strategy, and prioritize the needs of vulnerable populations worldwide, including children, those in poverty and conflict zones, women and girls, and marginalized communities.[76] Psychiatrists can write letters or emails, call or leave voicemails for their representatives, or write articles supporting legislation like the MINDS Act, extending their advocacy reach.

With a little time and effort, physician advocates can identify emerging or proposed legislation or existing laws that move them personally—either as prospective policies to implement or as destructive policies to reform or abolish—by visiting the Web sites of their local, state, or federal legislators, or by joining with the existing legislative advocacy arms of their professional organizations. The APA and AACAP offer online resource centers and host national "advocacy days" yearly in Washington, DC, providing education and structure for interested advocates to engage.

SUMMARY

In 2021, the AAP, the AACAP, and the Children's Hospital Association announced a National Emergency in Child and Adolescent Mental Health, commenting on the unprecedented escalation in psychiatric need and pediatric safety risk in the time of the COVID-19 pandemic.[77] As the nation's emergency rooms witness a surge in children grappling with mental health issues and a shortage of health care professionals to attend to them, the impact may be felt disproportionately on a vulnerable and marginalized population already burdened by discriminatory policies, inadequate health care infrastructure, language and cultural barriers, limited health literacy, and stigma in many forms.[78,79]

Effectively addressing the barriers to mental health care for migrant children requires a comprehensive approach that considers their unique experiences throughout the migration and resettlement journey. It is crucial that advocates understand the social determinants of health that influence children's well-being and recognize the intricate interplay between governmental policies, health systems, community actors, and individual patient's unique circumstances and needs. Fortunately, promising practices are emerging within communities and inroads are being made in the legislative sphere, all of which are fundamentally powered by the immeasurable strength and resilience of migrant children and families themselves. Still, the challenges endure and the need for compassionate and determined advocates persists, beckoning physicians who might heed the call.

CLINICS CARE POINTS

- Individual-level advocacy in pediatric care for migrants involves considering the child, caregivers, and local support systems as interconnected elements of the child's functional circle, promoting well-being through both direct clinical advocacy and paraclinical advocacy, identifying health needs and bolstering resources beyond immediate clinical disease.

- It is important to recognize implicit bias and approach care and advocacy efforts with a framework of cultural humility and accountability.

- Practicing advocacy on behalf of migrant children's mental health requires clinical agency that extends beyond the traditional scope of care, collaborating with interdisciplinary partners and overcoming systemic barriers to support culturally inclusive and equitable health care delivery.

DISCLOSURE

The authors have nothing to disclose.

REFERENCES

1. Verhagen IL, Noom MJ, Lindauer RJL, et al. Mental health screening and assessment tools for forcibly displaced children: a systematic review. Eur J Psychotraumatol 2022;13(2):2126468.
2. Vance MC, Kennedy KG, Wiechers IR, et al, editors. A psychiatrist's guide to advocacy. 1st edition. Washington, DC: American Psychiatric Association Publishing; 2020.
3. World Health Organization and Calouste Gulbenkian foundation. Social determinants of mental health. World health organization; Geneva, Switzerland, 2014. Available at: https://apps.who.int/iris/bitstream/handle/10665/112828/9789241506809_eng.pdf.
4. Cotton NK, Shim RS. Social determinants of health, structural racism, and the impact on child and adolescent mental health. J Am Acad Child Adolesc Psychiatry 2022;61(11):1385–9.
5. Castañeda H, Holmes SM, Madrigal DS, et al. Immigration as a social determinant of health. Annu Rev Publ Health 2015;36:375–92.
6. Gagnon M, Kansal N, Goel R, et al. Immigration status as the foundational determinant of health for people without status in Canada: a scoping review. J Immigr Minority Health 2022;24(4):1029–44.
7. Betancourt JR, Maina AW. The Institute of Medicine report "Unequal Treatment": implications for academic health centers. Mt Sinai J Med 2004;71(5):314–21.
8. Song SJ, Ventevogel P, editors. Child, adolescent and family refugee mental health: a global perspective. Switzerland: Springer Nature Switzerland AG; 2020.
9. Di Nicola V, Leslie M, Haynes C, et al. Clinical considerations for immigrant, refugee, and asylee youth populations. Child Adolesc Psychiatr Clin N Am 2022;31(4):679–92.
10. UNICEF. Child migration. UNICEF Data: monitoring the situation of children and women website 2021. Available at: https://data.unicef.org/topic/child-migration-and-displacement/migration/ Accessed May 27, 2023.
11. Wiechers IR, Pinals DA, Mauch DE, et al. Conceptualizing advocacy. In: Vance MC, Kennedy KG, Wiechers IR, et al, editors. A psychiatrist's guide to advocacy. 1st edition. Washington, DC: American Psychiatric Association Publishing; 2020. p. 17–30.
12. Dobson S, Voyer S, Hubinette M, et al. From the clinic to the community: the activities and abilities of effective health advocates. Acad Med 2015;90(2):214–20.
13. Luft LM. The essential role of physician as advocate: how and why we pass it on. Can Med Educ J 2017;8(3):e109–16.
14. Ugorji O, Vance MC, Bayner JS. How do I become and advocate?. In: Vance MC, Kennedy KG, Wiechers IR, et al, editors. A psychiatrist's guide to advocacy. 1st edition. Washington, DC: American Psychiatric Association Publishing; 2020. p. 57–78.
15. American Medical Association. Declaration of professional responsibility; San Fransisco, CA. 2001. Available at: https://www.ama-assn.org/delivering-care/public-health/ama-declaration-professional-responsibility.
16. Varkey B. Principles of clinical ethics and their application to practice. Med Princ Pract 2021;30(1):17–28.

17. Kennedy KG. Legislative advocacy. In: Vance MC, Kennedy KG, Wiechers IR, et al, editors. A psychiatrist's guide to advocacy. 1st edition. Washington, DC: American Psychiatric Association Publishing; 2020. p. 119–46.

18. Wilson FA, Stimpson JP. Federal and state policies affecting immigrant access to health care. JAMA Health Forum 2020;1(4):e200271.

19. Crookes DM, Stanhope KK, Kim YJ, et al. Federal, state, and local immigrant-related policies and child health outcomes: a systematic review. J Racial Ethn Health Disparities 2022;9(2):478–88.

20. Office of the High Commissioner for Human Rights. Convention on the rights of the child; New York, NY, By general assembly resolution 44/25. 1989. Available at: https://www.ohchr.org/en/instruments-mechanisms/instruments/convention-rights-child.

21. Stubbe Østergaard L, Norredam M, Mock-Munoz de Luna C, et al. Restricted health care entitlements for child migrants in Europe and Australia. Eur J Publ Health 2017;27(5):869–73.

22. Mousin CB. Rights disappear when US policy engages children as weapons of deterrence. AMA J Ethics 2019;21(1):E58–66.

23. Hill J, Rodriguez DX, McDaniel PN. Immigration status as a health care barrier in the USA during COVID-19. J Migr Health 2021;4:100036.

24. Vargas ED, Ybarra VDUS. Citizen children of undocumented parents: the link between state immigration policy and the health of Latino children. J Immigr Minority Health 2017;19(4):913–20.

25. Martinez O, Wu E, Sandfort T, et al. Evaluating the impact of immigration policies on health status among undocumented immigrants: a systematic review. J Immigr Minority Health 2015;17(3):947–70 [published correction appears in J Immigr Minor Health. 2016 Feb;18(1):288. Rhodes, Scott (corrected to Rhodes, Scott D).

26. Kaiser Family Foundation (KFF). 2022. Health coverage and care of immigrants. KFF. Available at: https://www.kff.org/racial-equity-and-health-policy/fact-sheet/health-coverage-and-care-of-immigrants/. Accessed May 27, 2023.

27. Markkula N, Cabieses B, Lehti V, et al. Use of health services among international migrant children - a systematic review. Glob Health 2018;14(1):52.

28. Beier J, Fredricks K. A path to meeting the medical and mental health needs of unaccompanied children in U.S. Communities. Washington, DC: Migration Policy Institute and American Academy of Pediatrics; 2023.

29. National Immigration Law Center. (2020). Understanding the impact of key provisions of COVID-19 relief bills on immigrant communities. National immigration law center. Available at: https://www.nilc.org/issues/economic-support/impact-of-covid19-relief-bills-on-immigrant-communities/. Accessed May 28, 2023.

30. Hacker K, Anies M, Folb BL, et al. Barriers to health care for undocumented immigrants: a literature review. Risk Manag Healthc Pol 2015;8:175–83.

31. Jaiswal J. Whose responsibility is it to dismantle medical mistrust? future directions for researchers and health care providers. Behav Med 2019;45(2):188–96.

32. United States code, 2006 edition, supplement 4, Title 42 - the public health and welfare. Available at: https://www.govinfo.gov/app/details/USCODE-2010-title42/USCODE-2010-title42-chap6A-subchapII-partG-sec265 . Accessed May 27, 2023.

33. Pillai D, Artiga S. Title 42 and its impact on migrant families. KFF. 2022. Available at: https://www.kff.org/racial-equity-and-health-policy/issue-brief/title-42-and-its-impact-on-migrant-families/. Accessed May 27, 2023.

34. Hampton K, Heisler M, Pompa C. Neither safety nor health: how Title 42 expulsions harm health and violate rights. PHR. 2021. Available at: https://phr.org/our-work/resources/neither-safety-nor-health/. Accessed May 28, 2023.

35. Isacson A. 10 things to know about the end of Title 42. WOLA. 2023. Available at: https://www.wola.org/analysis/end-title-42/. Accessed May 27, 2023.

36. Song SJ. Mental health of unaccompanied children: effects of U.S. immigration policies. BJPsych Open 2021;7(6):e200.

37. Koss D, Sagot A. Advocacy for children and families. In: Vance MC, Kennedy KG, Wiechers IR, et al, editors. A psychiatrist's guide to advocacy. 1st edition. Washington, DC: American Psychiatric Association Publishing; 2020. p. 217–31.

38. Pumariega AJ, Rothe E, Mian A, et al. Practice parameter for cultural competence in child and adolescent psychiatric practice. J Am Acad Child Adolesc Psychiatry 2013;52(10):1101–15.

39. Hall WJ, Chapman MV, Lee KM, et al. Implicit racial/ethnic bias among health care professionals and its influence on health care outcomes: a systematic review. Am J Public Health 2015;105(12):e60–76.

40. Severe J, Riba M, Tasman A. Advocacy for immigrants, refugees, and their families. In: Vance MC, Kennedy KG, Wiechers IR, et al, editors. A psychiatrist's guide to advocacy. 1st edition. Washington, DC: American Psychiatric Association Publishing; 2020. p. 217–31.

41. Williams JC, Vance MC, Budde KS. Patient-level advocacy. In: Vance MC, Kennedy KG, Wiechers IR, et al, editors. A psychiatrist's guide to advocacy. 1st edition. Washington, DC: American Psychiatric Association Publishing; 2020. p. 81–95.

42. Panter-Brick C, Grimon MP, Eggerman M. Caregiver-child mental health: a prospective study in conflict and refugee settings. J Child Psychol Psychiatry 2014;55(4):313–27.

43. Slobodin O, de Jong JT. Family interventions in traumatized immigrants and refugees: a systematic review. Transcult Psychiatr 2015;52(6):723–42.

44. Fazel M, Betancourt TS. Preventive mental health interventions for refugee children and adolescents in high-income settings. Lancet Child Adolesc Health 2018;2(2):121–32.

45. Lee T, Fouras G, Brown R. American Academy of Child and Adolescent Psychiatry (AACAP) Committee on Quality Issues (CQI). Practice parameter for the assessment and management of youth involved with the child welfare system. J Am Acad Child Adolesc Psychiatry 2015;54(6):502–17.

46. Fiscella K, Sanders MR. Racial and ethnic disparities in the quality of health care. Annu Rev Publ Health 2016;37:375–94.

47. Mangrio E, Sjögren Forss K. Refugees' experiences of healthcare in the host country: a scoping review. BMC Health Serv Res 2017;17(1):814.

48. Lax Y, Cohen G, Mandavia A, et al. Landlord behavior after receiving pediatrician-generated letters to address poor housing conditions. JAMA Netw Open 2021;4(10):e2128527.

49. Shier G, Ginsburg M, Howell J, et al. Strong social support services, such as transportation and help for caregivers, can lead to lower health care use and costs. Health Aff 2013;32(3):544–51.

50. Potvin LA, Fulford C, Ouellette-Kuntz H, et al. What adults with intellectual and developmental disabilities say they need to access annual health examinations: system navigation support and person-centred care. Can Fam Physician 2019; 65(Suppl 1):S47–52.

51. Rey-Casserly C, McGuinn L, Lavin A, COMMITTEE ON PSYCHOSOCIAL AS-PECTS OF CHILD AND FAMILY HEALTH, SECTION ON DEVELOPMENTAL AND BEHAVIORAL PEDIATRICS. School-aged children who are not progressing academically: considerations for pediatricians. Pediatrics 2019;144(4). e20192520.

52. Sullivan AL, Simonson GR. A systematic review of school-based social-emotional interventions for refugee and war-traumatized youth. Rev Educ Res 2016;86(2): 503–30.

53. United States Department of Agriculture. Child nutrition programs. Available at: https://www.fns.usda.gov/cn . Accessed May 27, 2023.

54. Youth.gov information website. Afterschool Programs. Available at: https://youth. gov/youth-topics/afterschool-programs . Accessed May 27, 2023.

55. Ferdowsian H, McKenzie K, Zeidan A. Asylum medicine: standard and best prac-tices. Health Hum Rights 2019;21(1):215–25.

56. Gartland MG, Ijadi-Maghsoodi R, Giri M, et al. Forensic medical evaluation of chil-dren seeking asylum: a guide for pediatricians. Pediatr Ann 2020;49(5):e215–21.

57. Ferrera MJ, Giri M. What should count as best practices of forensic medical and psychological evaluations for children seeking asylum? AMA J Ethics 2022;24(4): E267–74.

58. Lustig SL, Kureshi S, Delucchi KL, et al. Asylum grant rates following medical evaluations of maltreatment among political asylum applicants in the United States. J Immigr Minority Health 2008;10(1):7–15.

59. Office of the high commissioner for human rights. Istanbul Protocol: manual on the effective investigation and documentation of torture and other cruel, inhuman or degrading treatment or punishment, professional training series No. 8/Rev. 2; New York, NY. (2022). Available at https://www.ohchr.org/sites/default/files/ documents/publications/2022-06-29/Istanbul-Protocol_Rev2_EN.pdf.

60. Tyrer RA, Fazel M. School and community-based interventions for refugee and asylum seeking children: a systematic review. PLoS One 2014;9(2):e89359 [pub-lished correction appears in PLoS One. 2014;9(5):e97977].

61. Thomas MS, Crosby S, Vanderhaar J. Trauma-informed practices in schools across two decades: an interdisciplinary review of research. Rev Res Educ 2019 Mar;43(1):422–52.

62. Videvogel S, Verelst A. Supporting mental health in young refugees: a resilience perspective. In: Song SJ, Ventevogel P, editors. Child, adolescent and family refugee mental health. Switzerland: Springer Nature Swizterland; 2020. p. 53–65.

63. Duong MT, Bruns EJ, Lee K, et al. Rates of mental health service utilization by children and adolescents in schools and other common service settings: a sys-tematic review and meta-analysis. Adm Policy Ment Health 2021;48(3):420–39.

64. Gower S, Jeemi Z, Forbes D, et al. Peer mentoring programs for culturally and linguistically diverse refugee and migrant women: an integrative review. Int J En-viron Res Publ Health 2022;19(19):12845.

65. Snider L, Hijazi Z. UNICEF community-based mental health and psychosocial support (MHPSS) operational guidelines. In: Song SJ, Ventevogel P, editors. Child, adolescent and family refugee mental health. Switzerland: Springer Nature Swizterland; 2020. p. 101–19.

66. Kotter JP. Leading change: why transformation efforts fail. Boston, MA: Harvard Business Review Press; 1997.

67. Li L, Franklin T. Organizational advocacy. In: Vance MC, Kennedy KG, Wiechers IR, et al, editors. A psychiatrist's guide to advocacy. 1st edition. Wash-ington, DC: American Psychiatric Association Publishing; 2020. p. 97–114.

68. Morrise L, Stevens KJ. Training patient and family storytellers and patient and family faculty. Perm J 2013;17(3):e142–5.

69. Friedman RA. The role of psychiatrists who write for popular media: experts, commentators, or educators? Am J Psychiatr 2009;166(7):757–9.

70. Pantti M, Ojala M. Caught between sympathy and suspicion: journalistic perceptions and practices of telling asylum seekers' personal stories. Media. Culture & Society 2019;41(8):1031–47.

71. Barron DS, Budde KS, Gold JA, et al. Engaging the popular media. In: Vance MC, Kennedy KG, Wiechers IR, et al, editors. A psychiatrist's guide to advocacy. 1st edition. Washington, DC: American Psychiatric Association Publishing; 2020. p. 191–209.

72. Osipov R. Healing narrative-ethics and writing about patients. Virtual Mentor 2011;13(7):420–4.

73. World Health Organization. Advocacy for mental health; Geneva, Switzerland. 2003. Available at: https://apps.who.int/iris/handle/10665/333227.

74. Dreier H. Alone and exploited, migrant children work brutal jobs across the U.S. February 25, 2023. Available at: https://www.nytimes.com/2023/02/25/us/unaccompanied-migrant-child-workers-exploitation.html. Accessed April 11, 2023.

75. U.S. Department of Labor. Departments of Labor, Health and Human Services announce new efforts to combat exploitative child labor. DOL. 2023. Available at: http://www.dol.gov/newsroom/releases/osec/osec20230227. Accessed May 28, 2023.

76. Congress.gov website. S.2105 - MINDS Act. Available at: https://www.congress.gov/bill/117th-congress/senate-bill/2105/all-info and H.R.3988 - MINDS Act. Available at: https://www.congress.gov/bill/117th-congress/house-bill/3988 . Accessed May 27, 2023.

77. American Academy of Pediatrics. AAP-AACAP-CHA declaration of a national emergency in child and adolescent mental health. 2021. Available at: https://www.aap.org/en/advocacy/child-and-adolescent-healthy-mental-development/aap-aacap-cha-declaration-of-a-national-emergency-in-child-and-adolescent-mental-health/. Accessed May 28, 2023.

78. AACAP. Severe Shortage of child and adolescent psychiatrists illustrated in AACAP Workforce Maps. 2022. Available at: https://www.aacap.org/aacap/zLatest_News/Severe_Shortage_Child_Adolescent_Psychiatrists_Illustrated_AACAP_Workforce_Maps.aspx . Accessed May 28, 2023.

79. Lebrun-Harris LA, Ghandour RM, Kogan MD, et al. Five-year trends in US children's health and well-being, 2016-2020. JAMA Pediatr 2022;176(7):e220056 [published correction appears in JAMA Pediatr. 2022 Apr 4;:null] [published correction appears in JAMA Pediatr. 2023 Mar 1;177(3):323].

Trauma Informed Best Practices and Resiliency

Jeanette M. Scheid, MD, PhD

KEYWORDS

- Immigration • Asylum • Children • Development • Trauma-informed

KEY POINTS

- Children and youth experiencing the immigrant/asylum process will have experienced trauma that will impact their emotions and behavior.
- Children's developmental stages will affect their responses to the immigrant/asylum experiences and associated traumatic exposures.
- Child and adolescent psychiatrists can use both their knowledge of child development and trauma-informed care principles when working with children, youth, and families.
- Child and adolescent psychiatrists should use their knowledge and expertise to advocate for environments that support health, safety, and resiliency.

INTRODUCTION

Children who experience fleeing from their home countries, whether with family members or unaccompanied, will likely have experienced trauma in their home country[1] and possibly in government custody.[2] The specific circumstances will be different for each child, as well as its impact on their sense of safety and wellbeing. The response of caring systems should remain grounded in the known principles of trauma-informed care, an understanding of best practices based on evidence-based and informed principles, culturally responsive interventions, and the developmental process. In addition, care providers should be working to maximize the safety of the environment in which they are interacting with children and youth and considering the style, approach and content of each interaction to balance the purpose of the interaction with the safety and security needs of each child or youth. In doing so, it will be possible to address multiple needs ranging from basic care and support to diagnosis and treatment to determining eligibility for asylum.

PRINCIPLES OF TRAUMA-INFORMED CARE

The Substance Abuse and Mental Health Services Administration's Trauma and Justice Strategic Initiative (2014)[3] defined the concept of trauma as resulting from event(s)

Michigan State University, 909 Wilson Road B119, East Lansing, MI 48824, USA
E-mail address: scheid@msu.edu

Child Adolesc Psychiatric Clin N Am 33 (2024) 181–191
https://doi.org/10.1016/j.chc.2023.09.005
1056-4993/24/© 2023 Elsevier Inc. All rights reserved.
childpsych.theclinics.com

or circumstances experienced by the individual as physically or emotionally harmful or life threatening and having lasting adverse effects on functioning and well-being. The initiative identified 4 key assumptions to drive trauma informed care systems (**Fig. 1**) and defined 6 key principles defining a trauma-informed approach to care (**Fig. 2**). These principles will be reflected throughout the suggestions for approaching children and families in this article.

The National Child Traumatic Stress Network (NCTSN) has developed and collected an array of materials that health care practitioners, including child and adolescent psychiatrists, can use as they prepare to work with children and youth affected by immigrant and refugee-related trauma (see Refugee Trauma Section in references).[4] These range from a formal report of the American Psychological Association Presidential Task Force on Immigration to a story of the impact of traumatic stressors on a Guatemalan immigrant family to an exploration of mandated reporting in the context of immigration to a resource focusing on bridging and collaboration among refugee-serving and children's services providers.

The definitions, assumptions, and principles summarized earlier should be integrated not only into individual clinical contacts between children/youth and child and adolescent psychiatrists but also as child and adolescent psychiatrists consult with agencies in developing programs intended to support children and youth who are immigrants seeking asylum and safety. Subsequent sections of this article outline practical approaches for this integration across a range of clinical and consultative encounters.

DEVELOPMENTAL TASKS AND IMPACT OF IMMIGRANT/REFUGEE TRAUMA
Infants

Infants require nearly constant attention from a limited number of dedicated caregivers who provide adequate responses to the limited variety of basic needs, that is, feeding, changing, and soothing. This attention promotes the achievement of the primary developmental tasks of building attachments and acquiring the capacity for basic regulation of daily routine that form the building blocks of learning trust and cause and effect and developing emotional awareness and regulation.

We know from developmental neuroscience as reviewed by Van den Bergh and colleagues (2020)[5] that even prior to delivery, maternal stress can make children more vulnerable to gaps in developing self-regulation and challenge their capacity to respond as expected to usual caregiving. Children involved in refugee/asylum settings may also experience developmental challenges.[6] When working with parent-infant

Assumptions when Developing Trauma Informed Care Systems

- **Realizes** impact of trauma and recovery
- **Recognizes** the signs and symptoms of trauma
- **Responds** through policy, procedure and practice
- **Resists** re-traumatization

Fig. 1. Assumptions when developing trauma informed care systems.[3]. (Reference 3: Substance Abuse and Mental Health Services Administration. SAMHSA's Concept of Trauma and Guidance for a Trauma-Informed Approach. HHS Publication No. (SMA) 14-4884. Rockville, MD: Substance Abuse and Mental Health Services Administration, 2014)

Principles of Trauma Informed Care Approach

- Safety
- Trustworthiness/transparency
- Peer support
- Collaboration and mutuality
- Empowerment/voice/choice
- Recognition of culture, history and gender issues

Fig. 2. Principles of trauma informed care approach.[3]. (Reference 3: Substance Abuse and Mental Health Services Administration. SAMHSA's Concept of Trauma and Guidance for a Trauma-Informed Approach. HHS Publication No. (SMA) 14-4884. Rockville, MD: Substance Abuse and Mental Health Services Administration, 2014)

dyads in the setting of immigration, refugee, and asylum services, it is important to ask about the prenatal period, screen for developmental and intellectual disorders, refer for formal assessment as needed, and provide education to parents about the possibility that the infant may be more reactive and irritable than expected even though their caregiving is appropriate.

Because infants may also be impacted by other risks, including family members with developmental disorders, or other prenatal exposures including parental substance use, it will be important to inquire about these exposures, recognizing the importance of doing so in a manner that is both generally culturally sensitive and also aware of how the information gathered may impact the immigration or asylum process at the family level and child protection law in the local jurisdiction.

Teams working in settings where parents who are caring for infants in short term refugee/asylum settings need to advocate for an environment that provides the capacity to regulate lighting, to limit noise, and to maximize privacy. Child and adolescent psychiatrists working in these settings should engage parents in discussions about family history and prenatal circumstances, perinatal events, and parents' observations of their infant. If the child and adolescent psychiatrist is less comfortable providing general psychiatric services, it may be necessary to advocate for access to a broader team including general psychiatry and/or substance use services providers who can support parents. Finally, teams providing ongoing care regardless of setting should have information about the child's history as gathered by previous healthcare providers and should be alert to indications of delays in achieving developmental milestones.

If infants have been separated from their parents they must have access to a small number of attentive caregivers. Under these circumstances the infants are likely to be especially stressed, so a quiet, calm environment will be particularly important to fostering safety. Early in separation if infants have been breast fed, it will be important to be attentive to any impact from change to formula feeding.

Toddlers

The chief tasks for toddler age children are to use the secure attachment platform and basic self-regulation achieved in infancy to engage in a broader exploration of their environment and work toward additional self-control including toilet training and responding to appropriate correction or direction. They will still need frequent opportunities to return to their trusted caregivers during their explorations.

Toddlers experiencing the disruption of immigration and asylum are likely to lose some of the developmental milestones they may have achieved at least for a time. Children who have been toilet trained may have bowel and bladder incontinence, and those who have generally been sleeping well may have difficulty falling asleep or sustaining sleep and may experience nightmares or night terrors even if they haven't had these before. Children perceived to be clingy and anxious or more irritable may actually be seeking safety and connection.

Understanding the child's developmental course to date, the family environment/stressors prior to the immigration/refugee process, and the time frames of the family's immigration and asylum journey are critical to understanding the context of any current difficulties. It will be important to provide education to parents/caregivers that when children are stressed it is normal for them to lose capacities for some period and typical for them to regain these capacities with time, care, and support.

When possible, advocating for an organizational structure that recognizes parents' primary role as their child's safe haven and providing them the support to engage effectively based on their culture and experience should limit the impact of the traumatic events to the extent possible. This support, including access to formal early childhood mental health resources, should be maintained throughout the process of immigration and when settling into a new home and community.

When children are separated from parents, they are more likely than children who remain with parents to experience sleep, emotional, and behavioral disturbances more intensely and for a longer period of time. Other explanations for sleep disturbances should also be assessed as soon as possible during the immigration process because healthy sleep is important to development and wellbeing.[7] Alternative caregivers should be made aware of the child's history, should be provided the resources they need to provide attentive caregiving, and should be part of a team engaged in ongoing assessment and treatment to ensure that the child regains age-appropriate functioning.

Young Children

Preschool-age children are focused on navigating the rules of engagement with parents and reinforcing their sense of family roles and relationships. This is the work necessary to move into the broader world of school and peer relationships comfortably. Children who are experiencing immigration/seeking asylum with their families are attempting to accomplish these developmental tasks in a setting where the broader family system is stressed and may not be able to reflect usual family roles. Even when children's experiences up to this point have not been traumatic, the stresses related to immigration will likely result in some regression that may include irritability and limit testing as well as anxiety-driven challenges to restful sleep. If children are separated from their parent(s) at this stage, the loss of security arising from familiar parental relationships will increase their distress.

In this age group, children may be able to describe their experiences and emotions more clearly than possible for younger children. Treating teams should afford the space for this exploration first and provide age-appropriate reflection and support based on the child's report. This may include formal treatment of trauma-related symptoms and other sources of distress.

As is true of younger children, the family unit should be maintained if possible. Teams should work with organizations to provide family space together. Parents should be supported in maintaining their parenting style and family routines like eating and sleeping. When children are separated from their parents, new caregivers need as much information as possible about the child. Any known issues that could affect health, emotions, and behavior should be provided and caregivers provided the support to address these.

School-Age Children

In the best of circumstances children in this group would be positioned through successful completion of earlier developmental stages to be comfortable spending a large part of every day with peers and teachers and having a solid home base they can return to at the end of the day. It is also in the school setting that even children without exposure to significant trauma may demonstrate emotional, behavioral, and/or learning issues. The circumstances related to immigration, refugee, and asylum-seeking[2] may increase this risk. It is unlikely that parents will have records of their children's academic progress from their country of origin. Language may provide an additional barrier to communication about this history. Finally, children who have attended school and engaged in peer relationships in their home country communities are likely to experience a sense of loss and disconnection from their home culture.

When children are with their parents, the family unit should remain the home base and source of support and cultural grounding. Parents are also the best source of information about their child's prior health and mental health history, their schooling, and their past social environment. Children who have been separated from parents may be able to provide some of this information, though their ability to do so will depend on their level of distress. Caregivers in any environment should focus first on creating an environment with as much safety and comfort as possible while caregivers and other team members attempt to obtain information from the child and other sources. Services and supports, including those related to school access, should be established as efficiently as possible early on and maintained throughout the asylum process. School systems can provide a valuable source of supports and routines to children throughout their immigration journey.

Adolescents and Young Adults

Youth in this age group are more likely to be unaccompanied and will have had variable experiences related to their history of family relationships. If they did experience nurturing family relationships, then they may have an age-appropriate sense of self that can provide a reserve under the circumstances of their immigration/refugee journey. If they also have some means of regular contact with family members, they can use this as an additional source of support. When youth and their families were under sustained stress in their home country prior to attempting immigration/asylum, these stressors, perhaps going back to early childhood, will be a burden the youth carries,. It is also possible that the youth will have experienced family/relational trauma aside from those related to the immigration process and may or may not have had any opportunity to obtain support or treatment. As it is normative for adolescents to exercise more independence, youth may not appear interested in family support. If they have been used to fending for themselves, they may brush off attempts to engage supportive adults including family. Youth in these circumstances will also be working through cultural identity issues that may affect their functioning.[8,9] As it will likely be true that unaccompanied youth will be in temporary housing with other youth, teams working with adolescents should advocate both for age-appropriate privacy consistent with the youth's cultural experience and for age-appropriate peer-to-peer interaction time.

Teams working with unaccompanied youth should determine their sources of support, whether family and friends in their origin country or family/relatives/new communities of support in the United States, and arrange for contact as frequently as possible. Consider inviting supports to appointments, following the Trauma Informed Care principle of peer support. These same supports may prove to be a source of historical information about the youth that will help with developing a plan of care over the intermediate and long term. Second, it will be important to identify factors outside of language barriers that impact the youth's capacity to engage in the assessments that are needed, whether clinical assessment for the purpose of diagnosis and treatment, or an assessment to determine eligibility under asylum rules. Third, those working with children and families need to be aware that children's stress may be affected by their parents' legal status in a similar fashion to those who have grown up with an undocumented parent.[10,11] This could include a stated or perceived responsibility for finding employment to contribute to the family's financial needs. Addressing these barriers early will enhance the ability of helping teams to meet the youth's needs.

In summary, child and adolescent psychiatrists have the training and experience in child and adolescent development, the impact of family relationships, and the impact of exposure to trauma that provides a firm platform from which to draw as they approach trauma-informed care with immigrant and refugee children, youth, and families. This knowledge and skill can and should be brought to bear both as clinicians and as advocates. In approaching this work, child and adolescent psychiatrists should refresh their understanding of trauma-informed principles and practices generally and the specific circumstances characterizing the immigrant and refugee experience. Resources to do so are listed at the end of this article.

ENVIRONMENT: HOW TO SET UP FOR CONNECTIONS AND CONVERSATIONS
Setting

The physical settings in which most children adolescents and families are waiting for immediate decisions about their next steps are far from ideal for any kind of encounter intended to learn more about the issues facing a child or adolescent. Conditions may be crowded, and there may be limited privacy. There may be little in the way of age-appropriate toys or other activities to engage the child when the focus is on parents or to use to engage the child when they are the focus of an interview.

Individuals working in these settings should advocate for devoting some space and basic materials to support assessments, including comfortable chairs for adults, child sized tables and chairs, and some way to shield the space both from outside noise and from those outside the space hearing the assessment conversations. Chairs should also be moveable to allow for children and family members to arrange seating that will maximize their comfort, addressing both safety and empowerment/voice/choice.

Plain paper along with coloring books or sheets reflecting a range of age needs along with crayons, markers, and pencils should be provided. If possible, a white board with markers should be available either for children to write/draw or to support dialog between the clinician and the child/family, increasing transparency. Clinicians should have access to any commonly used screening or assessment questionnaires written in the languages likely to be used by the people in these settings. Finally, because children and youth may need breaks during an assessment, there should be a room close by that can be supervised appropriately but is also comfortable and where calming items can be made available.

Interviewer Body Language

Interviewers need to be aware of their body language. Being able to sit comfortably in an open posture, but also to shift to more alertness and focus is important. It is also important to be aware of body language in the context of history, culture, and gender. Children may benefit from the opportunity to engage in playful interactions, and if the assessment is being done in a setting where more than one child is present, being aware of and responding appropriately to other children may increase parent and child engagement. Prior to engaging in an interview, it will be important to inquire about and prepare for specific cultural norms for interaction, including whether to engage in frequent direct eye contact, who should be approached first when multiple family members are in the room, and whether and/or how to engage individual children or adolescents separately from their families. The NCTSN resources may be useful here, as would peer support. Interviewers can also ask children and families directly about their cultural norms and responding to this information addresses transparency and empowerment. In the heightened stress of immigration/refugee/asylum settings the clinician will need an additional level of awareness of these issues and be able to flexibly adjust their posture and approach when children and/or families show escalated distress. For example, attempts to engage in playful interactions with children that may be typical in most settings may not be perceived as safe under these circumstances, so acute awareness of responses to such overtures are necessary. Asking about children's usual interactions with peers and adults and in different settings can improve the clinician's capacity to be respectful during interactions.

Interviewer Spoken Language

Another barrier to communication in immigration/refugee settings will likely be related to language. Any clinician engaging in assessments of any kind who is not fluent in the primary language used by the child and family should have an interpreter present who is fluent in that language. An interpreter should have some training in the assessment process and in the boundaries of their role. Clinicians unfamiliar with using interpreter services may need to do some background preparation as well so that they are equipped to set up the interview space correctly and engage the child and family members directly through body language and eye contact. Although family members or other informal contacts sometimes offer to serve as interpreters, and may be the only option for focused assessments in emergency circumstances if unable to access professional interpreters, they should not provide interpretation for full psychiatric assessments, especially when the primary goal or some aspect of the assessment relates to asylum status eligibility.[11]

Once primary language barriers are addressed, clinicians engaging children, youth, and families in addressing any health, behavioral health or legal status issues should screen for developmental barriers to communication including expressive/receptive language disorders, reading difficulties that may impact the capacity to complete any requested rating scales, or any challenges to non-verbal communication that may impact interview findings.

Along with identifying and addressing developmental barriers to communication, the interviewer must consider the impact of the individual's emotional state on information gathering throughout any interview process. The issues that need to be explored will vary depending on the purpose of the interaction, as will be discussed later, but as suggested by O'Brien (2016) beginning the interview with more neutral topics and building some degree of rapport before exploring more substantive issues may allow the child and their parents to reduce initial anxiety and engage more successfully.[12] During the early parts of an interview, the clinician can also introduce the possibility that difficult topics may be discussed, normalize shifts in emotional state, and provide concrete information about the steps that the child and/or family can take to address discomfort during the interview, including taking a break or using resources like a calming space and then returning to the interview process.

UNDERSTANDING AND NAVIGATING THE SHIFTING GOALS OF INTERACTION

Clinicians working with children and families involved with immigration, asylum, or refugee related services may be called upon to engage in various interactions. Some of these, for example, determining eligibility for asylum, have very specific requirements and need specific training/expertise. Others, including providing general emotional support in detention settings, conducting a clinical assessment, or guiding level of care recommendations, are more driven by individual goals. If a child and family are involved in assessments for different purposes over time, the goals and processes of different assessments may overlap, and information obtained from one interaction may inform others. Understanding factors that affect disclosure of life stories, for example, those documented by van Os and colleagues,[13] including children's mistrust as a barrier to disclosure and the interviewer's respectfulness and patience as a facilitator to disclosure, is important. From the standpoint of trauma-informed principles, specifically those *promoting safety, empowerment, and transparency*, being clear about how all information is used and stating that teams may use information obtained in some settings to inform other assessments may reduce the times that a child or family needs to provide the same information, especially information that is difficult to share.

Collaboratively determining the goal or extent of the assessment aligns with the principle of mutuality, empowerment/choice/voice. Assessments may need to be completed over multiple sessions.

Supporting Comfort

Supporting comfort may be the most common element all the interactions teams will have with children and families. At its most basic this involves ensuring that basic needs for food and shelter are met and supporting family time. Although these basic needs are often outside the direct control of a clinician, gaps in basic needs can be an area for consultation and advocacy with supporting systems.

During any interaction children and families may talk about life experiences, both good and bad. These disclosures are an opportunity to build an understanding of the child and the impact of all experiences on their emotions and well-being. It may also provide insight into the child's strengths including interests and strategies they use to calm distress. With the child's or parents' permission, these could be incorporated into other assessments including those to determine asylum eligibility to reduce the likelihood of retraumatization.

Supporting Asylum Evaluation

The process of assessing a youth for the purposes of asylum are well-defined and discussed in the literature. Asylum examinations should only be conducted by someone with appropriate training and experience. Engaging in the process of asylum determination is nearly certain to range from emotionally uncomfortable to significantly painful. Using some of the setting (privacy, place to take a break, and calm) and interaction (starting with less loaded topics and attentiveness to emotional reactions to content in discussion) strategies may make these difficult conversations more comfortable for the asylum seeker and more productive.

In addition to managing the interview process itself, it will be important to educate the child and family about possible distress and include time and space for the child and family to decompress after an asylum interview. This may include additional time in a quiet, calming space, returning to family if they are present, or engaging in any activity that they identify as enjoyable. It will also be important to alert anyone working with the child/adolescent to be made aware that they have engaged in an asylum interview so that the staff can be aware of any discomfort the child or adolescent may display in the days following the interview. If the youth is prone to anger outbursts or destructive behavior both the youth and the staff will need supports to reduce safety risks. Taking all these steps promotes safety and empowerment.

Supporting Diagnostic and Treatment Evaluation

As is true of asylum determination, there are guidelines and best practices for comprehensive diagnostic interviews and subsequent treatment planning. Clinicians working in this sphere should follow guidelines such as those provided by the American Academy of Child and Adolescent Psychiatry, including the historic Practice Parameters for the Psychiatric Assessment of Children and Adolescents (1997)[14] and other practice guidelines for assessment and treatment. In fact, one could argue that under these circumstances it is particularly important to think comprehensively about a child's strengths, needs, symptoms, and likely diagnoses. Accomplishing what is often a challenging task may be particularly difficult because of the realities of immigrationFor children with their families, parents should be sources of important information. For children not with their immediate families, it may be possible to reach families by phone, or to engage with extended family, especially if the family members are planning to provide ongoing supervision or support.

If a diagnostic interview is occurring in a context where an asylum interview has also occurred, and if it is possible to do so, the information from the asylum interview should be incorporated into the clinical interview and documentation. The interviewer could note the information mentioned in the asylum interview but focus on the thoughts, emotions, and behavior related to the experiences during the clinical interview. The documentation may be important to include in multiple sections of the clinical report including the history of present illness, medical history, social history, mental status examination, case formulation, and recommendations. If a diagnostic interview occurs before a planned asylum interview, the clinician will need to be aware of the limits of confidentiality and provide only the information that is possible under confidentiality rules, or obtain permission from the child and family to disclose information that may reduce the stress associated with the asylum interview.

As is true of an asylum interview, children may be distressed following a clinical interview as well. This potential can be normalized by the clinical provider, support can be offered, and staff working with the child and family can be engaged to provide support as the child settles back to some degree of calm.

Addressing Gaps in Access or Contact with Families

Throughout all the immigration processes for children/youth who are unaccompanied by parent(s) there should be efforts to maintain direct contact and to provide updates to both children and parents about the status of the other. There should be accommodations made to provide direct contact, preferably by video conferencing, although if this is not possible then telephone calls or any other means of connection should be used. Clinicians working with children will need to assess any safety concerns, including assessing for parental maltreatment, as a prerequisite to this planning.

Parents should be engaged in providing historical information for all levels of assessment whether considering how to provide basic needs and comfort, understanding factors that may impact the child's capacity to engage in assessments for any purpose and for collateral information related to both asylum and clinical assessments. If a clinical assessment results in any recommendations for medication intervention, parents should be engaged to provide this consent, although there may be local and regional law, policies, and rules to allow teams to provide treatment if it is not possible to engage parents. Similar to any of the evaluation processes that occur with children and families, interpreters should be engaged so that treatment recommendations can be explained adequately, and parents can provide informed consent. It is especially important to engage caregivers about their reservations about medication and to try and understand their own ideas about how to support the child.

SUMMARY: PUTTING IT ALL TOGETHER–BUILDING A FULL UNDERSTANDING OF THE CHILD/YOUTH

Throughout a time that children and their families are engaged in detention or other formal "holds", whether families are separated or together, the goals should be to provide immediate support for basic health and well-being needs, to engage in appropriate information gathering for a variety of purposes from asylum requests to diagnostic evaluations, to engage in treatment when needed, and to use all interactions efficiently and transparently to maximize the benefits of the assessment and to minimize and mitigate the distress that such evaluations may cause.

The information obtained during these early parts of the child's and family's immigration journey should also be documented well and forwarded on to subsequent teams in the broader systems of care including caregivers, health providers, mental health providers, schools, and community supports so that the ongoing needs of the child and family can be identified and addressed in the context of their story. Doing so will provide the best likelihood that children and families will be successful in their journey.

CLINICS CARE POINTS

- Using existing knowledge of child development is key to providing and advocating for the optimal environment for migrant children and families.
- Following trauma informed principles: safety, trustworthiness/transparency, peer support, collaboration and mutuality, empowerment/voice/choice, and recognition of cultural historical and gender issues should guide all interactions with migrant children, youth, and families.
- When possible use interactions and information obtained for one purpose for other migrant and asylum needs to minimize traumatic exposures.

DISCLOSURE

No commercial financial disclosures. The author provides non-clinical consulting services under contract between Michigan Department of Health and Human Services and Michigan State University as part of faculty duties.

REFERENCES

1. Thomas S, Thomas S, Nafees B, et al. 'I was running away from death' – the preflight experiences of unaccompanied asylum seeking children in the UK. Child Care Health Dev 2004;30(2):113–22.

2. Kronick R, Rousseau C, Cleveland J. Asylum-seeking chilren's experiences of detention in Canada: a qualitative study. Am J Orthopsychiatry 2015;85(3): 287–94.
3. Substance Abuse and Mental Health Services Administration. SAMHSA's concept of trauma and guidance for a trauma-informed approach. HHS publication No. (SMA) 14-4884. Rockville, MD: Substance Abuse and Mental Health Services Administration; 2014.
4. NCTSN – Refugee Trauma (https://www.nctsn.org/what-is-child-trauma/trauma-types/refugee-trauma).
5. Van den Bergh BRH, van den Heuvel MI, Lahti M, et al. Prenatal developmental origins of behavior and mental health: the influence of maternal stress in pregnancy. Neurosci Biobehav Rev 2020;117:26–64.
6. Morinaga M, Rai D, Hollander A-C, et al. Migration or ethnic minority status and risk of autism spectrum disorders and intellectual disabiliity: systematic review. Eur J Publ Health 2020;31(2):304–12.
7. Mindell JA, Williamson AA. Benefits of a bedtime routine in young children: sleep, development, and beyond. Sleep Med Rev 2018;40:93–108.
8. Patel SG, Bouche V, Thomas I, et al. Mental health and adaptation among newcomer immigrant youth in United States educational settings. Current Opinion in Psychology 2023;49:101459.
9. Cowden JD, Kreisler K. Development in children of immigrant families. Pediatr Clin 2016;63:775–93.
10. Sidhu SS, Song SJ. Growing up with an undocumented parent in America: psychosocial adversity in domestically residing children. J Am Acad Child Adolesc Psychiatr 2019;58(10):933–5.
11. Levy J, Using an interpreter in psychiatric practice, *Carlat Child Psychiatry Report*, 11(5&6), 2020, 3-4.
12. O'Brien KH, Schlechter A. Is talking about what's wrong necessarily right: a positive perspective on the diagnostic interview. J Am Acad Child Adolesc Psychiatr 2016;55(4):262–4.
13. van Os ECC, Zijlstra AE, Knorth EJ, et al. Finding keys: a systematic review of barriers and facilitators for refugee children's disclosure of their life stories. Trauma Violence Abuse 2020;21(2):242–60.
14. King RA, Work Group on Quality Issues. Practice Parameters for the psychiatric assessment of children and adolescents. J Am Acad Child Adolesc Psychiatr 1997;36(10 Suppl):4S–20S.

Trauma Exposure in Migrant Children

Impact on Sleep and Acute Treatment Interventions

Beverly J. Bryant, MD

KEYWORDS

- Sleep • Trauma exposure • Migrant youth • Interventions

KEY POINTS

- Sleep disturbances in children are common and can have multiple etiologies, including trauma exposure or unfamiliar/uncomfortable residential or congregate care settings.
- There are no FDA-approved medications for pediatric PTSD or sleep disturbance.
- Psychological First Aid can be administered in the acute setting.
- Untreated sleep disturbances can be linked to suicidal ideation and self-harm.
- Of the medications available to treat acute sleep disturbances in trauma-exposed youth, prazosin, alpha-2 agonists, and trazodone seem to be first line from a clinical perspective.

INTRODUCTION

Disordered sleep is common in trauma-exposed youth. Nightmares, difficulties with sleep onset, disrupted sleep, and reduced quality of sleep occur in many children and adolescents who have experienced trauma, both directly and indirectly. The severity of the sleep disturbance is often linked to the proximity to the trauma.[1] For example, studies of children living near the World Trade Center during the 9/11 attacks found that those exposed to "high intensity" events, such as observing people jumping out of windows, seeing the towers collapse, and so forth, were more likely to have sleep difficulties than those who were not.[1] Likewise, migrant children have varying degrees of proximity to trauma, for example, witnessing violence toward family and friends and/or experiencing violence directly.

Sleep disruption can negatively affect neurobehavioral functioning, mood, learning, and academic performance.[2,3] Insufficient sleep has been linked to increased emotional dysregulation, difficulties with abstract reasoning, and even suicidal behavior.[4,5] Ongoing sleep disruption in youth can have both short- and long-term

Child Psychiatry, Talkiatry, 1400 N Coit Road #302, McKinney, TX 75071, USA
E-mail address: Beverly.bryant@talkiatry.com

Child Adolesc Psychiatric Clin N Am 33 (2024) 193–205
https://doi.org/10.1016/j.chc.2023.08.001
1056-4993/24/© 2023 Elsevier Inc. All rights reserved.

childpsych.theclinics.com

effects, including aggression, anger, irritability, and self-injury as well as increased risk for developing substance abuse disorders, elevated blood pressure, and reduced academic performance.[2,4-6] Unidentified sleep disturbances can also lead to misdiagnosis of disorders such as attention deficit disorder (ADHD) and mood disorders.[7] Sleep difficulties are linked to both hyperarousal and reexperiencing symptoms of posttraumatic stress disorder (PTSD),[4] and unresolved sleep problems potentiate other symptoms of PTSD.[1]

Much of the literature regarding disordered sleep in PTSD centers around adults and studies in pediatrics is limited.[5,8] In terms of psychopharmacology for disordered sleep, most studies have been conducted on non-traumatized youth.[2,6,9-12]

There are no federal drug administration (FDA)-approved medications for childhood PTSD, and medication is not the first-line recommended treatment.[13-16] Evidence-based trauma-focused psychotherapeutic interventions are far more effective, but not always readily available.[16] Children and adolescents in shelter situations may benefit most from supportive interventions such as Psychological First Aid[17] but may need medication to help them with acute sleep problems associated with their trauma. In spite of the urgent need, little has been written to inform clinical practice in this area. There are few randomized controlled trials, and much of the evidence is based on case reports, open label trials, retrospective chart reviews, and clinician opinion.[1,4,14,15,18-21] Some of the available evidence for the use of various medications will be reviewed.

BACKGROUND

It is estimated that 25% of children experience sleep problems at some point. Sleep patterns also change with development (**Fig. 1**), with a progressive decline in sleep duration within a 24-h period from birth to adolescence.[2,9] Daytime sleep (napping) decreases sharply between 18 months and 5 years.[2] Nightmares and sleep terrors occur in toddlers more often than older children so symptoms must be put into a developmental context.[2] Various studies report the prevalence of nightmares in non-traumatized youth to range from 6.8% to 20%, with slightly higher numbers

Infants (1–12 mo)	14–15 h/24 h at 4 mo and 13–14 h/24 h at 6 mo. Sleep periods last 3–4 h during first 3 mo, 6–8 h by 6–12 mo. 2–4 h naps twice a day between 6–12 mo.
Toddlers (12–36 mo)	12 h/24 h. Naps 0.5–3.5 h per day in one or two naps. By 18 mo, most give up the second nap.
Preschool children (3–5 y)	11–12 h/24 h. Most give up napping by age 5 with 25% continuing to nap at age 5. Cultural factors may play a role.
Middle childhood (6–12 y)	10–11 h/night. High levels of physiologic alertness during the day.
Adolescence (12–18 y)	Optimal 9–9.25 h/night. At onset of puberty, may develop as much as a 2-h sleep/wake phase delay (later sleep onset and wake times).

Fig. 1. Normative sleep patterns for age. (Owens JA. Pediatric Insomnia. *Sleep Medicine Clinics*. 2006;1(3):423-435. doi:https://doi.org/10.1016/j.jsmc.2006.06.009.)

for sleep disturbances such as difficulty falling asleep, waking up during the night, and daytime fatigue.[1] Numerous studies of trauma-exposed youth show the prevalence of nightmares to range from about 9% up to 80% depending on the type of trauma. These children also have higher rates of the other sleep difficulties described above.[1]

It would be interesting to know if developmental differences exist between older and younger children suffering from trauma-related sleep disturbances, but little data are available. Children who experience war conflict report nightmare prevalence from 13% to 40%.[1] Children who are not directly involved with the traumatic event may also experience sleep disruption. In a study by Pynoos and colleagues, 159 children ages 5 to 13 years reported symptoms on the PTSD-reaction index (RI) self-report after a sniper attack on the school playground.[1] Nightmares were reported in 62.9% of the children who were on the playground, 55.6% of children at the school, and 41.5% of children who were not at the school. Rates of sleep disturbance were higher, affecting 77.1% of the children on the playground, 55.6% of students at the school, and 48.8% of students who were not at the school that day.[1] In a study of 412 children from the Gaza strip, 80.8% reported distressing dreams and 63.6% reported sleep difficulty.[1] Variations in prevalence rates may be due in part to differences in study design.[1]

Other sleep problems such as sleep-disordered breathing and periodic limb movement, also occur in traumatized youth.[1] Adults with PTSD have less slow wave sleep, higher REM density, and more stage 1 sleep than controls.[1] There is evidence that sleep problems in youth can be predictive of later problems such as depression and anxiety in adulthood and adolescence.[1]

Changes in sleep architecture have been demonstrated by polysomnography in children with anxiety.[1] In one study, children with anxiety disorders had less slow wave sleep, greater sleep onset latency, and an increased number of awakenings than controls or children with depression.[1] Polysomnographic studies of children with PTSD are difficult to do, but studies using actigraphy have demonstrated that children with PTSD tend to have significantly higher sleep onset latencies and nocturnal activity than controls.[1] Almost all studies of pediatric PTSD and sleep disorders rely on subjective measures, which do not provide detailed information about the clinical presentation in these children.[1] Although actigraphy can provide estimates of sleep efficiency, it does not provide a measure of the bio-parameters necessary to diagnose many sleep disorders.[1]

Longitudinal studies have suggested that sleep problems in early childhood may increase the risk of developing stress-related psychiatric and behavioral disorders later in life, indicative of a possible bidirectional relationship.[1,6] In adults, sleep disruption predicts the severity and onset of PTSD symptoms.[1]

NORMATIVE SLEEP PATTERNS AND CHARACTERISTICS OF PEDIATRIC INSOMNIA

Normative sleep patterns change from infancy to adolescence as seen in **Fig. 1**.[22]

According to a national study of normative trends in sleep duration in 13 to 32 year olds, sleep duration is "developmentally patterned from adolescence through early adulthood." However, it also varies based on age, sex, race, and ethnicity.[22]

In their review article on pediatric insomnia, Veeravigrom and Chonchaiya[12] identify three components of pediatric insomnia.

1. Ongoing difficulty with sleep
2. Sufficient sleep opportunity
3. Difficulties with daytime function

Likewise, the investigators discuss the "3P" model of pediatric insomnia.[12]

1. Predisposing factors (ie, underlying medical or psychiatric conditions, age, sex, genetic predisposition, and temperament)
2. Precipitating factors (ie, acute traumatic events, PTSD, parent conflict)
3. Perpetuating factors (ie, inadequate sleep environment, poor sleep hygiene, and environmental pressures).

Migrant and refugee children suffer in all of these areas. The challenges of overcoming symptoms due to medical conditions (such as COVID-19), psychiatric conditions (such as bereavement and depression), acute traumatic events, and the difficulties of sleeping in a strange environment (such as a shelter), all contribute to sleep problems for these children. Numerous sleep problems have been identified related to the COVID-19 pandemic for both children and adults.[23] Whenever possible, the underlying factors contributing to the insomnia should be identified and addressed. Treatment of underlying medical conditions and/or making adjustments in the sleep environment may resolve the issue. On the other hand, trauma exposure has a direct impact on sleep.[12]

THEORIES FOR ETIOLOGIES FOR SLEEP DEPRIVATION IN TRAUMA-EXPOSED YOUTH

Differences in sleep architecture, differences in presentation of symptoms and developmental differences occur in disordered sleep patterns after exposure to trauma. Numerous theories have been developed to explain why exposure to trauma can affect sleep.[2] These theories are summarized by Giannakopoulos and Kolaitis in "Sleep problems in children and adolescents following traumatic life events" in *World Journal of Psychiatry,* 2021 February 19; 11(2): 27 to 34, as follows.[4]

Biological Theory

Increased levels of arousal and decreased activity in the areas of the brain that promote sleep onset may occur with traumatic stress. Sleep onset problems are quite common in traumatized children. Increased activity in the amygdala and decreased activity of the medial prefrontal cortex lead to increased physiologic arousal, which hinders sleep onset. Problems with sleep initiation must be distinguished from problems with sleep maintenance.

Safety and Attachment Theory

Naturally, the ability to sleep is related to a sense of safety. Imminent threat or perceived imminent threat may result in a desire to remain continuously alert and on guard. For children and adolescents, this can influence the development of a safe attachment style.

Emotional Memory and Affect Theory

This theory hypothesizes that sleep disturbances such as nightmares have a direct impact on emotional load and distress. Thus, increased frequency and severity of nightmares is associated with an increase in highly reactive emotional states.

Threat Simulation Theory

It is postulated that because actual threats occur during wakefulness, there is a heightened activation of the threat stimulation system. This leads to an increase in the recurrence and severity of threat experienced in dreams. The dreams reenact "the cognitive mechanisms needed for adequate threat perception and threat avoidance." Some studies have shown that the higher the level of severity of the traumatic event, the higher number of dreams, particularly threatening dreams, result.

Emotional Regulation Model

This model is based on the idea that traumatized individuals develop a fear network that contains fear-related information in the memory. Traumatic reminders result in a fear response and the need to defend oneself or flee. This level of hyper-alertness during sleep may lead to the traumatic dream being replayed over and over again in sleep.

Hyperarousal-Based Theory

This theory proposed that exposure to trauma results in an increased level of awareness and a higher sensitivity to external factors. Traumatized individuals reexperience trauma-related cues in their cognitive world, resulting in physiologic arousal and undesirable emotions that interfere with sleep.

Anxiety Buffer Disruption Assumption

This theory suggests that fear results in an increased level of awareness and a more sensitive response to external events. It proposed that fear leads to the gathering of traumatic clues in the cognitive world and intrusive thoughts. Fear can also make all PTSD symptoms worse by preventing constructive examination of traumatic experiences.

Depressive-Like Pathophysiology and Cognitive Hyperactivation

Abnormalities related to severe depression, such as elevated cortisol levels near sleep onset, increased sleep latency, and dysregulation of REM sleep also contribute to significant sleep disturbance. Excessive worry, rumination, and automatic negative thoughts may also cause hyperarousal resulting in sleep disruption.

LINK OF SLEEP DISRUPTION TO SUICIDE RISK

Independent of comorbid psychiatric illness, chronic sleep disturbances and nightmares increase the risk of suicidal behavior and self-injury in both children and adults.[4–6,24] Sleep inefficiency and increased heart rate have also been associated with suicidality. In 2018, Chiu and colleagues found that for every 1 hour increase in sleep, the risk of the development of suicidal plans in adolescents drops by 11%.[25] Autonomic measures such as heart rate variability have been correlated with the severity of PTSD and risk for suicide.[5]

TREATMENT CONSIDERATIONS

The nature of dreams is poorly understood. In PTSD, nightmares can occur during both REM and non-REM sleep.[10] Medications that suppress REM sleep are also known to induce nightmares. Various theories exist as to why. However, many agents can be associated with increased nightmares, including nicotine, selective serotonin reuptake inhibitors (SSRIs), stimulant medications, benzodiazepines, and antipsychotics.[10] Even antiviral agents, antibiotics, and immunosuppressant drugs can be associated with nightmares.[10] This makes the effort to identify medications for trauma-related sleep disturbance all the more complicated.

As previously noted, safety is an important requirement for sleep. Psychological First Aid is the first intervention needed for migrant traumatized youth.[17] Psychological First Aid was developed from a collaborative effort between the National Child

Traumatic Stress Network and the veteran administration's (VA's) National Center for Posttraumatic Stress Disorder. Although there are few data specifically related to the effects of PFA on sleep, the hope is that by helping to reduce the overall levels of physiologic arousal, normative sleep patterns will be enhanced. The five basic principles are safety, calm, connectedness, self and community efficacy, and hope. The goals are to offer practical assistance for immediate needs and concerns and to help trauma survivors to establish connections with each other as well as external supports (**Fig. 2**). It is important to have as much predictability as possible and to help children understand what to expect in the following hours to days.[17] Whenever possible, having a bedtime routine with calming and culturally relevant activities before sleep (such as stories with a comforting theme, prayer, and reassurance). Breathing and other relaxation techniques can be useful (**Fig. 3**).

Generally speaking, cognitive behavioral therapy (CBT) has been a cornerstone of treatment for sleep disturbances for both adults and children with PTSD as well as for other underlying mental health disorders.[4,5,8,13–16,26,27] Other trauma-informed psychotherapeutic interventions include psychoeducation, relaxation techniques, reconditioning of bed and bedroom as being conducive to sleep, and removal of any stimuli that are traumatic reminders. CBT for insomnia (CBTi) has been found to be useful in adults and has been adapted for children.[7] The most useful component of CBTi in a shelter setting most likely involves relaxation techniques such as progressive muscle relaxation, deep breathing, and visualization. It is important to encourage practice of these techniques when patients are not trying to fall asleep.[7]

In adults, Image Rehearsal Therapy, Exposure, Relaxation, and Rescripting therapy as well as Eye Movement Desensitization and Reprocessing therapy have been used with success.[5] However, in the acute setting, such as a shelter, these therapies may not be readily available.

In general, the most information available regarding the safety and efficacy of medications for sleep disorders in children comes from the pediatric literature,[9] studies of parasomnias[28] or studies of PTSD in adults.[8] Disorders of arousal during childhood such as sleep terrors, confusional arousals, and sleep walking occur most often in childhood and are usually self-limited and benign.[28] Information about medications that are effective in the specific treatment of sleep problems for children with psychiatric disorders is also limited and most medications are used off-label. Surveys of clinicians in practice have reflected the popularity of certain classes of medication.[18] A survey of Canadian child and adolescent psychiatrists in 2020 indicated that their top choices were melatonin, trazodone, and quetiapine.[18] However, melatonin may be contraindicated for sleep disturbances in traumatized youth due to its tendency to enhance nightmares and its effects on puberty.[9,29] Some of the evidence base, such as it is, for the use of various medications in treating trauma-related sleep disturbances will be reviewed here.

Provide contact and engagement
Enhance safety and comfort
Aid stabilization (eg. calm overwhelmed, agitated, and distraught survivors)
Gather information and prioritize assistance to identify immediate needs and concerns
Offer practical assistance and information
Connect survivors to family, friends, neighbors, and other supports
Promote adaptive coping techniques
Link survivors to other services or resources

Fig. 2. Psychological First Aid core actions and objectives. (Used with permission from the National Center for Child Traumatic Stress; Brymer, M., Mooney, M., Gurlitz Holden, M., Griffin, D., & Louie, K. (2022). Psychological First Aid (PFA) Online. Los Angeles, CA, and Durham, NC: National Center for Child Traumatic Stress.)

| Let's practice a different way of breathing that can help calm our bodies down. |
| Put one hand on your stomach like this (demonstrate) |
| OK, we are going to breathe in through our noses. When we breathe in, we are going to fill up with a lot of air and our stomachs are going to stick out like this (demonstrate) |
| Then, we will breathe out through our mouths. When we breathe out, our stomachs are going to suck in and up like this (demonstrate) |
| We are going to breathe in really slowly while I count to three. I am also going to count to three while we breathe out really slowly. |
| Let's try it together. Great job!" [you can make a game out of it by blowing bubbles or blowing paper wads or cotton balls across the table.] |

Fig. 3. Teaching a breathing exercise to children. (Used with permission from the National Center for Child Traumatic Stress; Brymer, M., Mooney, M., Gurlitz Holden, M., Griffin, D., & Louie, K. (2022). Psychological First Aid (PFA) Online. Los Angeles, CA, and Durham, NC: National Center for Child Traumatic Stress.)

PRAZOSIN

Prazosin is an alpha-1 antagonist used for blood pressure and benign prostatic hypertrophy. Numerous studies in adults have demonstrated efficacy in reducing trauma-related nightmares.[8] Results are varied, with some reports indicating that higher doses are needed in adults with PTSD nightmares, sometimes up to 45 mg.[8] Its use in children has been less well investigated and mainly consists of case reports and retrospective chart reviews.[15,27]

Keeshin and colleagues[15] conducted a retrospective chart review of youth at a trauma clinic between 2014 and 2016 and found that prazosin was effective and relatively well tolerated. Of the 34 patients who were available for follow-up, 79% received trauma-focused CBT. The sample was 82% female, 76% of whom had a history of sexual abuse, and 65% had at least one other psychiatric disorder. The mean age was 13.4 ± 2.9 years and the mean duration of prazosin treatment was 10.2 ± 8.1 weeks. The prazosin dose range was 1 to 15 mg at night, with 35% of patients taking more than 5 mg per day. Change in symptom severity was evaluated with the University of California, Los Angeles (UCLA) PTSD Reaction Index. Improvement in sleep and nightmares was statistically significant over time ($P < 0.001$). The main side effects were dizziness (18%), anxiety (9%), and headaches (6%). Unfortunately, these kinds of data are not available for most of the medications described here.

Hudson and colleagues[27] evaluated a group of 42 inpatient children taking prazosin by retrospective chart review between January 1, 2017 and July 31, 2019 and also found it to be helpful with few side effects. The youth in this sample also engaged in trauma focused-cognitive behavioral therapy (TF-CBT) per hospital protocol. Improvement in nightmares occurred in 57.1% of the sample. The degree of improvement was estimated based on review of prescriber progress notes. There was no significant change in systolic or diastolic blood pressure before and after starting prazosin and 81% reported having no adverse effects. The average dose in this study was 1.05 mg. This sample too was predominantly female (83%) and white (76%)

It should be noted that most of the children in both of these reviews were undergoing TF-CBT, the "gold standard" of evidenced-based treatment for this population. It is hard to know the specific degree to which prazosin reduced the symptoms as there were no comparisons between those who were and were not engaging in TF-CBT. However, given the tolerability of prazosin (1–15 mg) in this population,[15] it seems to be a reasonable agent to try for acute management of traumatic nightmares. There is great need for double-blind placebo-controlled studies of prazosin in this age group.

PROPRANOLOL

Propranolol has been studied in open trials for regulation of hyperarousal symptoms in children with mixed results. It is also used for treatment of hypertension and it is a centrally acting long chain beta blocker.[16] It has been used for treatment of stage fright and performance anxiety, and it is thought to be most effective in managing ongoing hyperarousal symptoms.[16,30] One open-label study found improvement in PTSD symptoms with propranolol, but other studies have not.[16] Again, these studies were not controlled for concomitant treatment with TF-CBT.

ALPHA-2 AGONISTS

The centrally acting alpha-2 agonists have been studied for treatment of ADHD and other impulse control disorders in children and adolescents. Clinician reports,[20] case reports, and open-label studies[14,15,30,31] have found clonidine to be helpful in reducing nightmares in children, but more robust studies are lacking. In open-label studies, clonidine has been found to reduce hyperarousal symptoms, reenactment symptoms, and nightmares.[16] In other pediatric sleep disorders, clonidine has been found to be helpful with problems initiating sleep, especially in children who are also suffering from ADHD.[9] However, peak effects occur within 2 to 4 hours and it may not be as helpful in maintaining sleep. Even though clonidine is known to mildly decrease REM sleep, it has been reported to increase nightmares in some patients.[10] It can also cause rebound hypertension if abruptly discontinued, making it more difficult to use in shelter populations.

Guanfacine is also a centrally acting alpha-2 agonist that may reduce hyperarousal symptoms in trauma-exposed children.[14] Case reports[21] indicate that because of its longer half-life, it may be more helpful in maintaining sleep, although it tends to be less sedating than clonidine. Although guanfacine extended release may be helpful in reduction of reexperiencing, avoidant, and hyperarousal symptoms, many children do not report improvement in their nightmares.[16] However, guanfacine was well tolerated in most reports.[16]

ANTIDEPRESSANTS
Selective Serotonin Reuptake Inhibitors

There have been no studies directly assessing the efficacy of SSRIs specifically for sleep. Even though SSRIs are known to suppress REM sleep, they are known to increase nightmares in some cases.[5] There seems to be an increase in vivid dreaming and dream recall, showing that these symptoms may be independent of REM suppression.[10]

Although antidepressants such as SSRIs have demonstrated efficacy in the treatment of adult PTSD, their use in children are not recommended. Antidepressants may be helpful in the treatment of comorbid depression and PTSD as well as the sleep disturbances associated with both diagnoses. However, behavioral dysregulation and the potential for increased suicidal ideation in young people can be problematic in use of these agents in a shelter setting where follow-up may be uncertain.

Cohen and colleagues performed the only double-blinded placebo-controlled study of sertraline efficacy as an enhancement of TF-CBT,[26] but sleep was not specifically studied.

Trazodone

There are no controlled studies for the use of trazodone for trauma-related sleep disorders, even though survey data show that it is often used for pediatric insomnia.[5,18,30]

Boafo and colleagues surveyed 67 active child and adolescent psychiatrists in Canada on their views about the efficacy of various sleep medications for youth and their prescribing preferences. Melatonin was the top choice (83%), and trazodone was rated as a second choice (56%). Respondents also rated perceived efficacy of various medications as follows: melatonin (97%), trazodone (81%), and quetiapine (73%). Other agents such as doxepin, tricyclic antidepressants, zaleplon, zolpidem, and lorazepam were rarely used due in part to concerns about long-term safety and suitability for youth.[18]

Tricyclic Antidepressants

Robert and colleagues conducted a prospective, randomized, double-blind study of pediatric burn patients with acute stress disorder in 1999. The study compared the efficacy of imipramine versus chloral hydrate in this population and concluded that imipramine is more effective. However, the investigators urged caution due to potential cardiovascular side effects and drug interactions.[11] These concerns in addition to concerns regarding potential toxicity limit their use.[12,30]

Second-Generation Antipsychotics and Mood Stabilizers

Foa and colleagues report that uncontrolled trials and case reports have demonstrated some utility for risperidone and quetiapine in youth with PTSD. Case reports suggest that quetiapine (50–100 mg/day) provided improvements in dissociation, anxiety, depression, and anger over a 6-week period.[30] Quetiapine is listed as having "weak" evidence for use as a single drug for adults with PTSD in guidelines by the American Academy of Sleep Medicine.[5] Foa cautions that with "scant evidence as to their utility in PTSD symptoms per se," the atypical neuroleptics should be used for treatment refractory PTSD or for patients with comorbid psychotic symptoms.[30] Despite perceived efficacy[18,30] concerns about weight gain and the availability of other agents merit caution in their use.[16]

Likewise, there have been some reports that mood stabilizers such as carbamazepine may be effective in the treatment of pediatric PTSD.[14,16,30] Open-label trials and retrospective case series have suggested possible improvement of PTSD symptoms with divalproex and oxcarbazepine. Again, there are concerns about metabolic syndrome and the absence of controlled studies in children.[16]

Antihistamines

Antihistamines are among the most commonly prescribed medications for sleep in pediatrics.[9,12] They are readily available and rapidly absorbed.[9] Diphenhydramine, hydroxyzine, and cyproheptadine are often widely used.[12] Case reports have suggested efficacy for cyproheptadine for traumatic dreams,[19] but widespread evidence is lacking. Others report that antihistamines can cause drug-induced disordered dreaming and nightmares.[10] Also, there have been five infant fatalities due to diphenhydramine reported in a case series.[32]

Melatonin

Melatonin is a common agent for pediatric insomnia in psychiatric and nonpsychiatric settings.[9,18] It is classified as a neurohormone[29] secreted by the pineal gland in response to darkness.[9,29] There are some reports that melatonin can be associated with an increase in nightmares, although the mechanism for this is unknown.[29] Melatonin increases REM sleep, but as discussed earlier, the development of nightmares seems to be independent of REM sleep.[28]

Circadian rhythm disturbances in children may be responsive to melatonin and it can be effective in the reduction of sleep onset latency, but it is not as useful in maintaining sleep.[9] It is also not regulated by the Food and Drug Administration in the United States, so preparations vary in strength. Melatonin can reduce seizure potential in some patients, and long-term use can be associated with suppression of the hypothalamic-gonadal axis, contributing to precocious puberty.[9] When melatonin is used, it is often most useful to give it 2 hours before desired sleep onset rather than immediately before bedtime.[32]

Benzodiazepines and Hypnotics

The use of benzodiazepines is discouraged in the treatment of PTSD for adults as well as children.[8,30] Hypnotics such as zaleplon and zolpidem have not been adequately studied in children[9] and have been associated with problematic side effects in adults, such as sleepwalking and other parasomnias.[9]

DISCUSSION

Although the evidence for the presence of sleep disorders in trauma exposed youth is overwhelming, to date, there have been no prospective double-blind placebo-controlled studies of any pharmacologic agents specifically for sleep. Likewise, there are no FDA-approved pharmacologic treatments for PTSD in children.[8,16]

It is widely accepted that trauma-focused therapies, particularly TF-CBT, are far more efficacious than medications in the treatment of both adult and pediatric PTSD.[8,13–16,26] However, in acute situations (such as in a shelter situation), these treatments are not available. The limited literature that does exist on the treatment of sleep disturbances in trauma-exposed youth is based on case reports, retrospective chart reviews, clinician opinion, and adult studies.[1,4,14,15,18–21] The only prospective double-blind study of sertraline as an adjunct to TF-CBT did not demonstrate significant benefit.[26]

Of all the agents studied, prazosin seems to have the best evidence for efficacy,[15,27] although that evidence is limited. Child psychiatrists routinely use medications such as melatonin, trazodone, guanfacine, and clonidine for sleep disturbances in children,[9,18] but the efficacy in treating PTSD nightmares is mixed. Medications such as quetiapine are considered effective by many psychiatrists,[18] but the risks of metabolic syndrome and other side effects limit long-term use.[16] Antihistamines such as diphenhydramine and hydroxyzine have been used in acute settings,[9] but some patients report a worsening of traumatic nightmares.[10] It has been suggested that cyproheptadine might be beneficial for traumatic nightmares,[19] but evidence is extremely limited.

Melatonin and SSRIs have been known to make traumatic dreams worse, even though they have opposite effects on REM sleep.[9,19,29] The nature of dreaming is unclear and it seems that nightmare frequency and severity are independent of REM sleep.[19] Tricyclic antidepressants such as imipramine can be effective,[11] but the risk of cardiovascular side effects and overdose limits their utility in a noncontrolled setting.

Mood stabilizers also have risks of metabolic syndrome and are rarely useful in an acute setting.[16] Benzodiazepines and hypnotics are discouraged.[8,9,30]

It would seem that regulation and calming techniques may be the most effective treatments of trauma-related sleep disturbances, but again, it can be difficult to use them in acute settings. Psychological First Aid[17] is a useful prerequisite to any other intervention with traumatized youth, especially interventions that enhance relaxation and grounding once primary needs are addressed.[17] Attention must be given to factors that predispose, precipitate, and perpetuate sleep problems in children.[12]

Numerous theories exist as to the etiology of sleep disturbances in PTSD.[4] There is evidence of the bidirectionality of sleep problems in youth and the development of psychiatric illness, even in later life.[1,6]

SUMMARY AND FUTURE DIRECTIONS

Medication has never been the first-line treatment of PTSD.[8,13–16] If medication is to be used, thought must be given to safety of administration in uncontrolled settings, such as a shelter. Comorbid conditions, such as mood disorders and psychotic disorders, may inform decisions in choosing a pharmacologic agent for sleep disturbance in trauma-exposed youth.[14,16,30]

Ongoing sleep disturbance is associated with increased risks of suicide and self-injury as well as poorer academic performance.[1,4–6,24]

The use of medications for the treatment of sleep disorders in trauma-exposed children is off-label and considered experimental by the FDA. This information must be part of an informed consent process and medication should only be used if clinicians have a good rationale.

Much more research is needed to provide solid clinical guidelines for when to use medications in terms of efficacy and duration of treatment. Care must be taken to avoid overprescribing, especially of antipsychotics in populations of impoverished children and children of color.

Polysomnography is difficult to do in this population but could provide more objective data. It would be valuable to know more about developmental differences in children with trauma-related sleep difficulties as well as effective interventions for very young or neurodiverse children.

Given the risks of untreated sleep disturbance in children and evidence that sleep disturbance and particularly traumatic dreams can prolong and worsen the course of other PTSD symptoms, it is imperative that more effort is placed into scientific study of the risks and benefits of pharmacologic agents not the first line of treatment but prazosin, alpha-2 agonists, and trazodone are often used in clinical settings.

CLINICS CARE POINTS

- Sleep disturbances, especially nightmares are common in trauma-exposed youth.
- It is important to evaluate predisposing, precipitating, and perpetuating factors when evaluating sleep disturbances in children.
- Sleep difficulties have been associated with suicidality; for every 1 hour increase in sleep, the risk of the development of suicidal plans in adolescents drops by 11%.
- Psychotherapeutic interventions such as Psychological First Aid, Cognitive Behavioral Therapy for insomnia, relaxation techniques, and others can be helpful in the acute setting such as a shelter.
- Medications are not the first line of treatment but prazosin, alpha-2 agonists, and trazodone are often used in clinical settings. Use of these medications are off-label.

DISCLOSURE

Nothing to disclose.

REFERENCES

1. Kovachy B, O'Hara R, Gershon A, et al. Sleep disturbance in pediatric PTSD: current findings and future directions. J Clin Sleep Med 2013;9(5):501–10.
2. Owens J. Classification and epidemiology of childhood sleep disorders. Sleep Medicine Clinics 2007;2(3):353–61.
3. Sadeh A. Consequences of sleep loss or sleep disruption in children. Sleep Medicine Clinics 2007;2(3):513–20.
4. Giannakopoulos G, Kolaitis G. Sleep problems in children and adolescents following traumatic life events. World J Psychiatr 2021;11(2):27–34.
5. Weber F, Thomas W. The many faces of sleep disorders in post-traumatic stress disorder: an update on clinical features and treatment. Neuropsychobiology 2021;81:85–94.
6. Willis TA, Gregory AM. Anxiety disorders and sleep in children and adolescents. Sleep Medicine Clinics 2015;10(2):125–31.
7. Pelayo R. Tools to Help Kids and Teens Sleep Better. The Carlat Child Report 2021; (6,7): 1, 4, 5, 10.
8. Detweiler M, Pagadala B, Candelario J, et al. Treatment of post-traumatic stress disorder nightmares at a veterans affairs medical center. J Clin Med 2016;5(12):117.
9. Owens JA. Pediatric insomnia. Sleep Medicine Clinics 2006;1(3):423–35.
10. Pagel JF. Drugs, dreams, and nightmares. Sleep Medicine Clinics 2010;5(2):277–87.
11. Robert R, Blakeney PE, Villarreal C, et al. Imipramine treatment in pediatric burn patients with symptoms of acute stress disorder: a pilot study. J Am Acad Child Adolesc Psychiatr 1999;38(7):873–82.
12. Veeravigrom M, Chonchaiya W. Insomnia: focus on children. Sleep Medicine Clinics 2022;17:67–76.
13. Cohen J. Practice parameter for the assessment and treatment of children and adolescents with posttraumatic stress disorder. J Am Acad Child Adolesc Psychiatr 2010;49(4):414–30.
14. Drury S, Henry C. Evidenced-based treatment of PTSD in children and adolescents:: where does psychopharmacology fit? Findling R. Child Adolesc Psychopharmacol News 2012;17(3):1–8.
15. Keeshin BR, Ding Q, Presson AP, et al. Use of prazosin for pediatric PTSD-associated nightmares and sleep disturbances: a retrospective chart review. Neurology and Therapy 2017;6(2):247–57.
16. Keeshin B, Strawn JR. Pharmacologic considerations for youth with posttraumatic stress disorder. J Korean Acad Child Adol Psychiatr 2017;28(1):14–9.
17. Psychological First Aid Online. National Child Traumatic Stress Network. Accessed May 9, 2023. learn.nctsn.org/course/view.php?id=596.
18. Boafo A, Greenham S, Sullivan M, et al. Medications for sleep disturbance in children and adolescents with depression: a survey of Canadian child and adolescent psychiatrists. Child Adolesc Psychiatr Ment Health 2020;14(1).
19. Gupta S, Austin R, Cali LA, et al. Letter to the editor: cyproheptadine. J Am Acad Child Adolesc Psychiatr 1998;37(6):570–1.
20. Horacek HJ. Letter to the editor: extended-release clonidine for sleep disorders. J Am Acad Child Adolesc Psychiatr 1994;33(8):1210.
21. Horrigan JP. Letter to the editor: guanfacine for PTSD nightmares. J Am Acad Child Adolesc Psychiatr 1996;35(8):975–6.

22. Maslowsky J, Ozer E. Developmental trends in sleep duration in adolescence and young adulthood: evidence from a national US sample. J Adolesc Health 2014;54(6):691–7.
23. Kumar N, Gupta R. Disrupted sleep during a pandemic. Sleep Medicine Clinics 2022;17(1):41–52.
24. Zheng X, Chen Y, Zhu J. Sleep problems mediate the influence of childhood emotional maltreatment on adolescent non-suicidal self-injury: the moderating effect of rumination. Child Abuse Neglect 2023. https://doi.org/10.1016/j.chiabu.2023.106161.
25. Chiu HY, Lee HC, Chen PY, et al. Associations between sleep duration and suicidality in adolescents: a systematic review and dose-response meta-analysis. Sleep Med Rev 2018;42:119–26.
26. Cohen JA, Mannarino AP, Perel JM, et al. A pilot randomized controlled trial of combined trauma-focused CBT and sertraline for childhood PTSD symptoms. J Am Acad Child Adolesc Psychiatr 2007;46(7):811–9.
27. Hudson N, Burghart S, Reynoldson J, et al. Evaluation of low dose prazosin for PTSD-associated nightmares in children and adolescents. Mental Health Clinician 2021;11(2):45–9.
28. Proserpio P, Terzaghi M, Manni R, et al. Drugs used in parasomnia. Sleep Medicine Clinics 2018;13(2):191–202.
29. Guardiola-Lemaître B. Toxicology of melatonin. J Biol Rhythm 1997;12(6):697–706.
30. Foa E. Psychopharmacotherapy in children and adolescents in Sri Lanka Journal of Psychiatry. Ariyasinge D, Williams SS, eds. Sri Lanka Journal of Psychiatry. 2017;8(1):568-572. doi:.
31. Pfefferbaum B. A review of the past 10 years. J Am Acad Child Adolesc Psychiatry 1997;36(11):1503–11.
32. Pelayo R, Dubik M. Pediatric sleep pharmacology. Semin Pediatr Neurol 2008;15(2):79–90.

Posttraumatic Stress Disorder in Our Migrant Youth

Vanessa C. D'Souza, MD

KEYWORDS

- Migrant youth • Trauma • Posttraumatic stress disorder • Migration
- Structural competency

KEY POINTS

- Identifying and treating post-traumatic stress disorder (PTSD) for migrant youth requires a collaborative effort between several systems of care including health care, education, legal, and migrant youth.
- As a clinician, developing an understanding of the individual's migration journey and stressors along with diagnostic tools including the University of California Los Angeles PTSD Reaction Index can help us understand the severity of PTSD symptoms for migrant youth
- By incorporating structural competency into our approach for migrant youth with PTSD, we can reduce the stigma and isolation that develops during the different stages of migration.

BACKGROUND

One in 5 children in the United States has been identified as an immigrant or a child of immigrant parents. By 2050, based on the demographic trends, it is predicted that this will increase to 1 in 3 children in the United States.[1] Within the last 50 years, there has been a significant shift in immigration patterns with more individuals from Latin America, Asia, and Africa coming to the United States to seek refuge, new opportunities, or both.[2] Looking at a bigger scale, there are more than 35 million migrant youth aged between 10 to 24 years worldwide.[3] As a result, there is more recognition that these individuals have exposure to several disparities on entering their new community, including lack of education, barriers to health care, barriers to the immigration system, discrimination, racism, and acculturation. Thus, migrant youth are considered a particularly vulnerable population that often has an increased risk of exposure to multiple traumatic and adverse experiences in their life that could subsequently lead to

Department of Psychiatry and Psychology, Mayo Clinic, 200 1st Street Southwest, Rochester, MN 55905, USA
E-mail address: dsouza.vanessa@mayo.edu

Child Adolesc Psychiatric Clin N Am 33 (2024) 207–218
https://doi.org/10.1016/j.chc.2023.10.005
1056-4993/24/© 2023 Elsevier Inc. All rights reserved.

posttraumatic stress disorder (PTSD). Whether there is immigration, forced migration, resettlement, or displacement we recognize how this can lead to significant adversity and trauma throughout their migration journey, and adds to the complexity of migrant youth with PTSD.

In this article, we will focus on the prevalence of PTSD in migrant youth, the risk factors associated with PTSD, and evidence-based interventions for this population. Recognizing the importance of the unique challenges and experiences of migrant youth with PTSD have and providing evidence-based interventions with a culturally sensitive approach is vital to their well-being, overall functioning, and ability to develop resiliency.

DIAGNOSIS

The initial presentation of PTSD in migrant youth is often somatic symptoms leading to missed opportunities for prompt diagnosis and treatment. Somatic symptoms often include headaches, stomachaches, body aches, pain, fatigue, and sleep disturbance, which are the most distressing symptoms for migrant youth.[4] These individuals will often seek assessments from primary care providers including family medicine and pediatricians for somatic symptoms before seeking an assessment by a mental health provider. The diagnosis of PTSD in migrant youth is based on the same diagnostic and statistical manual of mental disorders, fifth edition, text revision (2023) (DSM-5-TR) criteria for all individuals with PTSD, where there is the presence of intrusion symptoms, avoidance symptoms, negative alterations in mood and cognition, and alterations in arousal and reactivity following the exposure to a traumatic event for at least 1 month.[5]

The key diagnostic criteria that must be met for migrant youth aged older than 6 years are exposure to actual or threatened death, serious injury or sexual violence through direct experience, witnessing in person, learning about trauma that occurred to a close relative or friend, or experiencing repeated or aversive exposures details of the traumatic event. The latter of the repeated or aversive exposure is not a diagnostic criterion for children aged 6 years and younger.[5] Intrusion symptoms include involuntary recurrent distressing memories, distressing dreams, dissociative reactions, psychological reactions that are intense or prolonged, physiologic reactions from internal and external cues related to the trauma. The avoidance symptoms of PTSD are evidenced by the individual's effort to avoid distressing memories, thoughts, or feelings and/or the individual's effort to avoid external reminders related to the trauma.[6] Negative alterations related to PTSD may present as poor memory, negative beliefs or expectations, distorted thoughts about the cause of the traumatic event, negative emotional states, detachment from others, and decreased interest in significant activities.[7] Finally, with PTSD, there are changes in arousal and reactivity including hypervigilance, self-destructive behaviors, difficulty with concentration, sleep disturbances and irritable behaviors, which can be exhibited by extreme tantrums in youth aged younger than 6 years.[5,8]

It can be challenging to identify these symptoms in migrant youth as cultural differences and language barriers may affect the expression and interpretation of PTSD symptoms. This also has led to clinicians having difficulty differentiating psychosis from PTSD with migrant youth in the past. It was previously evident among adult populations, as Fazel and colleagues (2005) found that among 7000 refugees who resettled in Western countries those who had dissociative symptoms of PTSD were initially misunderstood as symptoms of psychosis.[9] More recently, it has been recognized that there is systematic misdiagnosis of psychosis among minority ethnic groups including migrant youth in the United States.[10] This suggests that careful assessment of PTSD is important for migrant youth that considers cultural differences, language barriers, and different expressions of distress.

Because a clinician builds their diagnostic formulation for PTSD in migrant youth, it is also important to be mindful and keep a broad differential including adjustment disorder, anxiety disorders, obsessive-compulsive disorder, major depressive disorder, attention-deficit/hyperactivity disorder, personality disorders, functional neurobiological disorder, psychotic disorders, and traumatic brain injury.[11] Recognizing comorbidities related to PTSD is also an important part of the diagnostic process. Comorbidities for migrant youth may include depressive disorders, anxiety disorders such as separation anxiety disorder, substance use disorders, and oppositional defiant disorder.[12]

PREVALENCE

Overall, the prevalence of PTSD among immigrant and refugee youth varies. Several studies have outlined that 9% to 36% of migrants have been diagnosed with PTSD.[13] More specifically, refugee youth and youth seeking asylum had a prevalence rate of PTSD of 30% to 40%, which indicates a significantly increased risk for PTSD compared with nonmigrant youth of 3% to 6%.[14] The wide range in prevalence of migrant youth with PTSD is related to how these studies defined the population of migrant youth and their methodology including how PTSD was diagnosed. Nonetheless, the prevalence of PTSD is substantially high among migrant youth and is associated with substance use disorder and conduct disorder especially among adolescents.[15]

One study used the Mini-International Neuropsychiatric Interview for Children and Adolescents along with incorporating the youth's social history to diagnose PTSD.[16] This structured interview screened for DSM-IV psychiatric disorders and suicidality in children and adolescents, and provided a quantitative score that could be used to monitor treatment response over time.[17] The University of California Los Angeles PTSD Reaction Index (UCLA PTSD-RI) has been used in most of studies for migrant youth in various settings to evaluate symptoms of PTSD. The UCLA PTSD-RI uses a semistructured clinician interview that focuses on all the symptom clusters for PTSD and includes reexperiencing intrusive distressing memories of the traumatic event(s), avoidance, and hyperarousal symptoms. This screening tool has a high sensitivity and high specificity for detecting PTSD symptoms in youth aged 7 to 18 years, which provides diagnostic accuracy with DSM-5 criteria. There is also a version of the UCLA PTSD-RI that allows clinicians to assess children aged younger than 6 years. All the versions of the UCLA PSTD-RI for children and adolescents incorporate a parent/caregiver interview. We recognize that with unaccompanied minors the parent/caregiver portion may not be completed but nevertheless, the structured interview can help ensure symptoms of PTSD are not overlooked. In addition, the UCLA PTSD-RI is validated in multiple languages, which allows children and adolescents to complete the screener with less difficulty because it reduces barriers with language when identifying symptoms of PTSD.[18] It is important to note that a positive outcome from the UCLA PTSD-RI, where the cutoff score is above 35, does not provide a definitive diagnosis of PTSD but rather indicates the need for further evaluation and assessment by a mental health provider.[19] These screening tools are helpful as a starting point for clinicians but it is important to recognize that there is a substantial difference in the diagnostic criteria of PTSD in the DSM-IV compared with the DSM-5-TR that should be considered. This includes how trauma is defined and response to trauma as the DSM-IV included intense fear, horror, and helplessness, which is no longer present in the DSM-5-TR.[5,20] While we wait for future steps to update screening tools to incorporate the updated diagnostic criteria of PTSD, clinicians will need to review these screening tools carefully to ensure diagnostic accuracy.

DISCUSSION

There is an association with PTSD, anxiety, and depression for migrant youth with trauma experienced at different migration stages. These youth may have experienced potentially traumatic and adverse events in their countries of origin, during their migration journeys, and in their new communities. This includes conflicts involving war, displacement, loss of loved ones, physical and sexual violence, and exploitation. Several studies classify trauma and exposure to adverse childhood experiences for migrant youth based on their stage of migration, which includes premigration, migration, and postmigration. During the premigration stage, the youth may experience several stressors including extreme poverty, sexual and physical abuse, neglect, abandonment, interpersonal violence, kidnapping, and loss of family from death or even murder in their home environment. When Sidamon-Eristoff and colleagues (2022) looked at migration of youth from Mexico to the United States, they found that of the 84 migrant children aged from 1 to 17 years released from an immigration detention facility, almost all, 97.4%, had experienced at least one premigration traumatic event. This premigration trauma along with the duration of parent–child separation has a direct correlation with the severity of PTSD symptoms.[21]

As the migrant youth makes the journey to the host country, there is a risk of exposure to adverse events leading to migration trauma. These adverse events include starvation, desertion, physical abuse, sexual abuse, gang violence, extortion, kidnapping, and incarceration. Finally, postmigration trauma occurs after arriving in the host country when the youth may have difficulty with acculturation, family unification, placement into foster care, the legal system and possibly living with relatives whom they have had no previous relationship.[15] Migrant youth may be reluctant to disclose their traumatic experiences due to fear and possibility reality of retaliation, and feelings of shame and/or guilt.

Postmigration stressors include difficulty with finances, housing, the immigration system, language barriers, isolation, acculturation stress, and stigma. These stressors have been shown to significantly influence youth more compared with premigration and migration potentially traumatic and adverse events.[22] In other words, a heightened stress response occurs for subsequent stressors following sensitization from premigration and migration trauma.[23] This is related to how the chronicity of daily stressors has the potential to further deplete coping mechanisms and resiliency. Postmigration stressors with their physical and psychological responses seem to have a direct effect on mental distress as well as indirect effects preventing recovery, influencing their ability to maintain resiliency and exacerbating symptoms of trauma.[24]

Many migrant youths are considered a minority in their host country, which has led to them encountering racial and ethnic discrimination. This can be related to their historical background that might include forced migration, slavery, segregation, and institutionalized racism.[2] The individual may carry emotional and psychological scars from their ancestors' experiences, influencing their response to trauma and the development of PTSD symptoms.[25] Because these individuals share similar feelings of fear, loss, or cultural disconnection with their cultural group leading to increased vulnerability to postmigration stressors that can be considered trauma and its effects.[26] Clinicians need to work with the migrant youth to understand their language, historical background, and values of migrant youth. This may allow the clinician to become more aware of if there is historical trauma that needs to be considered with the diagnostic formulation and approach to treatment. This also emphasizes the importance of the clinician having curiosity and working to understand the full life experience of the migrant youth they work with to understand their historical background. This curiosity can be fostered by being mindful, taking a nonjudgmental stance, and being aware of knowledge gaps when providing care to migrant youth.[27]

The cumulative experience of trauma that occurs in childhood during the migration stages along with intergenerational trauma has a greater influence on stress-regulatory processes for children and adolescents affecting their development and growth compared with if these experiences had occurred in their adulthood.[28] This is related to the heightened plasticity of the brain during development.[29]

CONSIDERATIONS

Family separation still occurs during the migration journey despite the efforts that have been made in the United States by implementing the "Zero Tolerance" policy to limit separating children from their parents or caregivers when taken into United States Customs and Border Protection custody since 2018.[30] Especially for young children, separation from a parent or caregiver is traumatic and affects the child's stress response because there is no longer an external source that is trusted by the child for emotion regulation along with disruption of attachment.[31] This alters the child's amygdala-to-prefrontal cortical circuitry involved with emotion regulation leading to behavioral difficulties and emotional problems.[32] The length of parent–child separation is considered a strong predictor for the severity of PTSD in migrant youth who underwent forced separation at the United States–Mexico border.[21]

INTERVENTIONS

PTSD left untreated can have a significant influence on an individual and leave a long-lasting impact on their mental health, developmental trajectory, physical health, and social functioning. This also places migrant youth at higher risk for suicide.[33] However, with the appropriate interventions many migrant youths can heal from the symptoms of PTSD and live fulfilling lives in their new communities.

Most guidelines for PTSD recommend psychotherapy as the first-line treatment.[7] The goal of these psychotherapeutic interventions is allowing the child or adolescent to develop and maintain coping strategies. Coping strategies are considered a dynamic continuous process that an individual will use to address and manage stressors in their life.[34] Coping styles were initially described as emotional coping and problem-focused coping but have now expanded to reappraisal coping, avoidance coping, and sense of hope.[35] Coping strategies used by migrant youth have varied by population and migration journey. Goodman (2004) found that Somali unaccompanied refugee minors often used avoidant and reappraisal coping strategies to address the stress of war, migration, and resettlement. Suppression and distraction helped the refugee minors focus on survival while developing feelings of community provided protection through a sense of responsibility to help others.[36] However, the use of avoidance coping strategies, especially social isolation correlates with PTSD among Somali refugees and led to a blunted cortisol reactivity making acculturation challenging.[37] Latinx migrant youth have also used avoidance coping strategies after exposure to violence, which has led to the exacerbation of PTSD symptoms.[38] Thus, recognizing that avoidance coping strategies might be the initial response for migrant youth that exacerbate symptoms of PTSD and lead to substance use is significant. The recognition of these maladaptive coping skills if the first part of the intervention.

Migrant will need youth guidance and further support by clinicians and the community including family and their cultural groups to develop and reinforce coping strategies that build on their resiliency. Effective coping strategies should be tailored to the migrant youth's individual needs. This can include creative expression, social support, maintaining a structured routine, limiting exposure to triggers, maintaining a healthy lifestyle, grounding techniques, and maintaining cultural connections. Developing these effective coping strategies typically starts with using a psychotherapeutic treatment modality such as trauma-focused cognitive behavioral therapy (TF-CBT).

TF-CBT is the most studied intervention for children and adolescents with PTSD. TF-CBT allows the individual to develop an understanding of the traumatic experiences that occurred, challenge negative thoughts, manage distressing emotions, and develop coping strategies that replace maladaptive ones including avoidance strategies.[39] TF-CBT for children and adolescents considers the role of the caregiver and development of the child's emotion regulation and coping capabilities; it is often delivered in 12 to 16 outpatient treatment sessions. When looking at the effectiveness of TF-CBT for children and adolescents overall, it is considered a viable treatment that reduces symptoms of PTSD but it is less clear regarding whether associated behavior problems and symptoms of depression have been affected. This is based on a meta-analysis of 10 studies where the effect size ranged from medium (6 studies) to large (3 studies), defined by standardized mean differences of Cohen's $d \geq 0.40$ and $d \geq 0.75$, respectively.[40] Modifying TF-CBT to include immigration factors, mental health beliefs, and understanding of relationships has led to significant improvements for unaccompanied minors with PTSD primarily from Central America living in the United States based on self-reporting assessments provided.[41]

An alternative therapeutic intervention is narrative exposure therapy (NET), where the individual creates a narrative of their traumatic experiences in a safe and therapeutic environment. This therapeutic modality is often considered when the individual has experienced multiple or prolonged traumatic events. The clinician would need to consider the patient's developmental stage of the individual, complexity of the trauma history and therapeutic goals. NET has been shown to be effective with adult refugees. The current randomized controlled trials of NET for refugee and migrant youth are very limited but have been shown to be effective with regard to reducing symptoms of PTSD, mainly among adolescents.[42] Recognizing that there are a limited number of randomized controlled trials with small sample sizes for treatment interventions for migrant youth with PTSD makes it challenging for clinicians to determine if alternative therapeutic options will be beneficial for the individual because there is the risk of retraumatization.

Using psychotherapeutic treatment modalities as a school-based intervention could be beneficial for migrant youth, especially unaccompanied minors.[43] Because schools continue to be one of the primary providers of mental health services for children in the United States through social workers, ensuring services are available for migrant youth is necessary. Having mental health care accessibility through the education system has led to improvement in behaviors, social-emotional functioning, and academic achievement.[44] Not to mention, it may also eliminate some of the barriers that migrant youth experience when seeking mental health care including stigma, insurance coverage, and financial barriers.[43] However, it is important to recognize that the treatment setting should be patient's and family's preferences that is going to be readily accessible to them while limiting stigma and isolation.

It is also important to emphasize that other therapy modalities may need to be considered for migrant youth due to neurodevelopmental disorders that may be present or their age and level of development. In some cases, parent–child interaction therapy (PCIT) may be the most effective, not require any specific adaptations, and lead to improvement with dysregulated behavior, trauma symptoms, and caregiver stress.[45] PCIT is conducted in 2 phases (child-directed interaction and parent-directed interaction) that involves the clinician guiding and coaching the caregiver in real-time play situations with the child. This therapeutic modality is also effective in strengthening the child–caregiver relationship by providing positive attention skills and warmth.[46] PCIT has led to a reduction of externalizing and internalizing symptoms related to trauma in children aged 2 to 7 years, with a large effect size of Cohen's classification d = 0.86.[45] Another alternative therapeutic intervention is nondirective play therapy. The measures of effectiveness for reducing symptoms of PTSD in migrant youth are limited with this treatment modality. However, a case report demonstrated that a child with severe autism spectrum disorder can build a therapeutic relationship with the clinician.[47]

Medications are considered second-line treatment of PTSD, with most efficacy with 3 selective serotonin reuptake inhibitors including sertraline, paroxetine, fluoxetine, and one serotonin reuptake inhibitor: venlafaxine.[7] Medication cannot be used as a standalone treatment of PTSD but has been helpful when paired with a therapeutic intervention. Medication should be considered when there is significant impairment of the migrant youth's day-to-day functioning or there is not an adequate response to psychotherapy. Atypical antipsychotics such as risperidone or aripiprazole can be helpful with extreme agitation, severe dissociation, or anxiety. Prazosin, an alpha-1 adrenergic antagonist is often used for nightmares and sleep disturbances associated with PTSD. When using medications for treatment of PTSD in migrant youth, the benefits need to outweigh the risks and it can be paired with a psychotherapeutic intervention.[48]

FUTURE DIRECTIONS

PTSD is a significant mental health concern for migrant youth. These young people face unique challenges related to trauma, migration, and acculturation. However, we see variations in the prevalence of diagnosis and effective interventions based on the limited accessibility migrant youth have to mental health, especially those in low-resource areas. It is becoming more of a necessity today to take a closer look at how providers obtain and document migration and trauma history for migrant youth. Providing information and practice opportunities to health-care providers and educators about the role of self-reflection and self-critique, using Metzl and Hansen's (2013) components of structural competency, in developing a culturally sensitive practice for migrant youth with PTSD could change how we address diagnosis and treatment.[49] Structural competency is made up of 5 concepts: recognizing structures shaping clinical interactions, developing extra-clinical language, rearticulating cultural formulations, structural interventions, and developing structural humility.[49] Recognizing structures involves clinicians being able to realize the influence economic, political, and physical factors have on medical decisions.[49] The development of extra-clinical language fosters the inclusion of interdisciplinary practices within medical conceptualizations, creating a broader language.[49] Rearticulating cultural formulation involves having familiarity with values among cultural groups while appreciating how structural determinants of health are designed to affect certain cultural communities to create inequality.[49] Structural interventions involve observing what structures are in place influencing a medical decision and recognizing how it can be different.[49] Finally, developing structural humility is having critical awareness and recognizing the limitations of structural competency.[49] An example of how the concepts of structural competency can be applied to migrant youth with PTSD is shown in **Table 1**. The development of partnerships and collaboration between various systems of care including educators and health-care providers is vital for this patient population. These steps allow us to address PTSD in migrant youth, and we can help promote their overall well-being and integration into their new communities.

Promoting integration with the host country through various aspects including sports, education, religious workshops, and community groups while maintaining cultural traditions can help migrant youth develop a sense of safety and security.[12] Finally, there is a need for a call to action for advocacy to ensure migrating youth receive humane and appropriate treatment in the different settings including

Table 1
An example of how Metzl and Hansens' concepts of structural competency can be used with migrant youth with PTSD to help reduce barriers associated with diagnosis and treatment[49]

Core Structural Competencies	Examples for Providers Working with Migrant Youth with PTSD
Recognizing the structures	• Identifying postmigration stressors: legal limitations to obtaining work, housing, immigration system, education, language barriers, social isolation, and stigma can have a more profound effect on migrant youth with PTSD[22] • For example, cost of medication and appointments including co-pays need to be considered for migrant youth but should not prevent the clinician from providing appropriate care
Developing extra-clinical language	• Understanding the historical background, cultural values, and language of migrant youth and how structural determinants of health intersect with these to increase barriers • Familismo values (where the individual keeps close ties to immediate and extended family) has led to resilience for Mexican-descent adolescents in the United States but may come into conflict with the US medical practice of encouraging separation and independence of adolescents[50]
Rearticulating cultural formulations	• Providing a deeper understanding of the structural forces migrant youth must face to receive treatment of PTSD that are in addition to cultural preferences • Explicitly discussing the structural barriers as distinct from cultural practices can foster increase awareness, result in more effective problem solving, and reduce the risk of retraumatization
Structural interventions	• Intervening in structural determinants of health inequities • Diversifying ways to access care such as incorporating treatment into school systems beyond formal treatment practices by developing daily routines, and teaching curriculums about heritage that honors diverse cultural practices and historical experiences
Developing structural humility	• Having awareness as a provider of the evolving economic and structural issues migrant youth face with the legal system • Working with legal advocates to understand the legal needs and concerns for the migrant youth, if present

immigration facilities, schools, and outpatient clinics by removing immigration policies in the host country that can lead to further trauma exposure.[51]

SUMMARY

Migrant youth face many challenges along their migration journey that leads to an elevated risk for PTSD. Compared with children and adolescents with no migration history, migrant youth have a higher prevalence of PTSD in the United States. Recognizing cultural differences through structural competency and understanding the individual's migration journey helps reduce misinterpretation of somatic symptoms, and dissociative symptoms that have raised concerns for psychosis for migrant youth. Historical trauma and family separation along with premigration, migration, and postmigration stressors all have an impact on the child's ability to maintain resiliency. Currently, TF-CBT has been the most effective intervention for migrant youth. Having opportunities to use TF-CBT as a school-based intervention is promising in eliminating barriers to care. It is hopeful that further studies for migrant youth with PTSD will lead to improvements in interventions and help support ongoing advocacy efforts.

CLINICS CARE POINTS

- Utilizinga strengths-based approach for treatment can build on resiliency for migrant youth and their caregivers. This has had good outcomes that validate hardships while helping the individual and their family to explore their role in overcoming adversity.[52]
- Recognizing the various ways trauma manifests for the individual along their migration journey and using diagnostic tools including the UCLA PTSD-RI has limitations but is one of our only current effective means to diagnose PTSD among migrant youth.[53]
- Delaying diagnosis and interventions for migrant youth with PTSD can lead to the development of other comorbidities including substance use disorder, anxiety disorders, major depressive disorder, conduct disorder, and oppositional defiant disorder.
- Advocacy is needed not only in the health-care system for migrant youth but in educational and legal systems to reduce postmigration stressors.

DISCLOSURE

The author has no commercial or financial conflicts of interest or any funding sources to disclose.

REFERENCES

1. Council NR. From generation to generation: The health and well-being of children in immigrant families. 1998;
2. Pumariega AJ, Jo Y, Beck B, et al. Trauma and US minority children and youth. Curr Psychiatr Rep 2022;24(4):285–95.
3. Dick B, Ferguson BJ. Health for the world's adolescents: a second chance in the second decade. J Adolesc Health 2015;56(1):3–6.
4. Schweitzer R, Melville F, Steel Z, et al. Trauma, post-migration living difficulties, and social support as predictors of psychological adjustment in resettled Sudanese refugees. Aust N Z J Psychiatr 2006;40(2):179–87.

5. Association AP. Diagnostic and Statistical Manual of Mental Disorders. Diagnostic and Statistical Manual of Mental Disorders.

6. Williamson JB, Jaffee MS, Jorge RE. Posttraumatic stress disorder and anxiety-related conditions. Continuum 2021;27(6):1738–63.

7. Merians AN, Spiller T, Harpaz-Rotem I, et al. Post-traumatic stress disorder. Med Clin North Am 2023;107(1):85–99.

8. El-Radhi AS. Management of common behaviour and mental health problems. Br J Nurs 2015;24(11):588–90.

9. Fazel M, Wheeler J, Danesh J. Prevalence of serious mental disorder in 7000 refugees resettled in western countries: a systematic review. Lancet 2005;365(9467): 1309–14.

10. Morgan C, Knowles G, Hutchinson G. Migration, ethnicity and psychoses: evidence, models and future directions. World Psychiatr 2019;18(3):247–58.

11. Auxéméry Y. Post-traumatic psychiatric disorders: PTSD is not the only diagnosis. Presse Med 2018;47(5):423–30.

12. De Vargas C, Ibeanu I, Odom C, et al. Unaccompanied migrant children and their challenges: a reintegration model. Washington, DC: AACAP; 2020.

13. Close C, Kouvonen A, Bosqui T, et al. The mental health and wellbeing of first generation migrants: a systematic-narrative review of reviews. Glob Health 2016;12(1):1–13.

14. Daniel-Calveras A, Baldaquí N, Baeza I. Mental health of unaccompanied refugee minors in Europe: a systematic review. Child Abuse & Neglect 2022; 133:105865.

15. Cardoso JB. Running to stand still: trauma symptoms, coping strategies, and substance use behaviors in unaccompanied migrant youth. Child Youth Serv Rev 2018;92:143–52.

16. Veeser J, Barkmann C, Schumacher L, et al. Post-traumatic stress disorder in refugee minors in an outpatient care center: prevalence and associated factors. Eur Child Adolesc Psychiatr 2021;32(3):419–26.

17. Sheehan DV, Sheehan KH, Shytle RD, et al. Reliability and validity of the mini international neuropsychiatric interview for children and adolescents (MINI-KID). J Clin Psychiatry 2010;71(3):17393.

18. Kaplow JB, Rolon-Arroyo B, Layne CM, et al. Validation of the UCLA PTSD Reaction Index for DSM-5: a developmentally informed assessment tool for youth. J Am Acad Child Adolesc Psychiatry 2020;59(1):186–94.

19. Steinberg AM, Brymer MJ, Decker KB, et al. The University of California at Los Angeles post-traumatic stress disorder reaction index. Curr Psychiatr Rep 2004;6(2):96–100.

20. Pai A, Suris AM, North CS. Posttraumatic stress disorder in the DSM-5: controversy, change, and conceptual considerations. Behav Sci 2017;7(1). https://doi.org/10.3390/bs7010007.

21. Sidamon-Eristoff AE, Cohodes EM, Gee DG, et al. Trauma exposure and mental health outcomes among Central American and Mexican children held in immigration detention at the United States–Mexico border. Dev Psychobiol 2022;64(1): e22227.

22. Chase E, Rezaie H, Zada G. Medicalising policy problems: the mental health needs of unaccompanied migrant young people. Lancet 2019;394(10206): 1305–7.

23. Koss KJ, Mliner SB, Donzella B, et al. Early adversity, hypocortisolism, and behavior problems at school entry: a study of internationally adopted children. Psychoneuroendocrinology 2016;66:31–8.

24. Dangmann C, Solberg Ø, Andersen PN. Health-related quality of life in refugee youth and the mediating role of mental distress and post-migration stressors. Qual Life Res 2021;30:2287–97.
25. Brave Heart MYH, Chase J, Elkins J, et al. Historical trauma among indigenous peoples of the Americas: concepts, research, and clinical considerations. J Psychoact Drugs 2011;43(4):282–90.
26. Fortuna LR, Tobón AL, Anglero YL, et al. Focusing on racial, historical and inter-generational trauma, and resilience: a paradigm to better serving children and families. Child Adolesc Psychiatr Clin 2022;31(2):237–50.
27. Epstein RM. Mindful practice. JAMA 1999;282(9):833–9.
28. Cloitre M, Stolbach BC, Herman JL, et al. A developmental approach to complex PTSD: childhood and adult cumulative trauma as predictors of symptom complexity. J Trauma Stress 2009;22(5):399–408.
29. Ismail FY, Fatemi A, Johnston MV. Cerebral plasticity: windows of opportunity in the developing brain. Eur J Paediatr Neurol 2017;21(1):23–48.
30. Monico C, Rotabi K, Vissing Y, et al. Forced child-family separations in the South-western US border under the "zero-tolerance" policy: the adverse impact on well-being of migrant children (part 2). Journal of Human Rights and Social Work 2019;4:180–91.
31. Teicher MH. Childhood trauma and the enduring consequences of forcibly sepa-rating children from parents at the United States border. BMC Med 2018;16:1–3.
32. Gee DG, Gabard-Durnam LJ, Flannery J, et al. Early developmental emergence of human amygdala–prefrontal connectivity after maternal deprivation. Proc Natl Acad Sci USA 2013;110(39):15638–43.
33. Viner RM, Coffey C, Mathers C, et al. 50-year mortality trends in children and young people: a study of 50 low-income, middle-income, and high-income coun-tries. Lancet 2011;377(9772):1162–74.
34. Sandler IN, Wolchik SA, MacKinnon D, et al. Developing linkages between theory and intervention in stress and coping processes, 1997, Handbook of children's coping: Linking theory and intervention, New York, 3–40.
35. Jani J, Underwood D, Ranweiler J. Hope as a crucial factor in integration among unaccompanied immigrant youth in the USA: a pilot project. J Int Migrat Integrat 2016;17:1195–209.
36. Goodman JH. Coping with trauma and hardship among unaccompanied refugee youths from Sudan. Qual Health Res 2004;14(9):1177–96.
37. Matheson K, Jorden S, Anisman H. Relations between trauma experiences and psychological, physical and neuroendocrine functioning among Somali refugees: mediating role of coping with acculturation stressors. J Immigr Minority Health 2008;10(4):291–304.
38. Epstein-Ngo Q, Maurizi LK, Bregman A, et al. In Response to community violence: coping strategies and involuntary stress responses among Latino ado-lescents. Cult Divers Ethnic Minor Psychol 2013;19(1):38–49.
39. Thielemann J, Kasparik B, König J, et al. A systematic review and meta-analysis of trauma-focused cognitive behavioral therapy for children and adolescents. Child Abuse & Neglect 2022;134:105899.
40. de Arellano MAR, Lyman DR, Jobe-Shields L, et al. Trauma-focused cognitive-behavioral therapy for children and adolescents: assessing the evidence. Psy-chiatr Serv 2014;65(5):591–602.
41. Patel ZS, Casline EP, Vera C, et al. Unaccompanied migrant children in the United States: implementation and effectiveness of trauma-focused cognitive behavioral therapy. Psychol Trauma 2022. https://doi.org/10.1037/tra0001361.

42. Samarah EMS. Narrative exposure therapy to address PTSD symptomology with refugee and migrant children and youth: a review. Traumatology 2022. https://doi.org/10.1037/trm0000427.

43. Franco D. Trauma without borders: the necessity for school-based interventions in treating unaccompanied refugee minors. Child Adolesc Soc Work J 2018; 35(6):551–65.

44. Nadeem E, Jaycox LH, Kataoka SH, et al. Going to scale: experiences implementing a school-based trauma intervention. Sch Psychol Rev 2011;40(4): 549–68.

45. Pearl E, Thieken L, Olafson E, et al. Effectiveness of community dissemination of parent–child interaction therapy. Psychological Trauma: Theory, Research, Practice, and Policy 2012;4(2):204.

46. Vanderzee KL, Sigel BA, Pemberton JR, et al. Treatments for early childhood trauma: decision considerations for clinicians. J Child Adolesc Trauma 2019; 12(4):515–28.

47. Josefi O, Ryan V. Non-directive play therapy for young children with autism: a case study. Clin Child Psychol Psychiatr 2004/10/01 2004;9(4):533–51.

48. Xiang Y, Cipriani A, Teng T, et al. Comparative efficacy and acceptability of psychotherapies for post-traumatic stress disorder in children and adolescents: a systematic review and network meta-analysis. Evid Based Ment Health 2021; 24(4):153–60.

49. Metzl JM, Hansen H. Structural competency: theorizing a new medical engagement with stigma and inequality. Soc Sci Med 2014;103:126–33.

50. Piña-Watson B, Gonzalez IM, Manzo G. Mexican-descent adolescent resilience through familismo in the context of intergeneration acculturation conflict on depressive symptoms. Translational Issues in Psychological Science 2019;5(4): 326–34.

51. Oberg C, Kivlahan C, Mishori R, et al. Treatment of migrant children on the US southern border is torture. Pediatrics 2020;146(5):1–12.

52. Miller KK, Brown CR, Shramko M, et al. Applying trauma-informed practices to the care of refugee and immigrant youth: 10 clinical pearls. Children 2019;6(8). https://doi.org/10.3390/children6080094.

53. MacLean SA, Agyeman PO, Walther J, et al. Mental health of children held at a United States immigration detention center. Soc Sci Med 2019;230:303–8.

Management of Psychiatric Emergencies Among Migrant Youth in Institutional and Community Settings

Linda Chokroverty, MD[a,b,]*

KEYWORDS

- Psychiatric emergencies • Behavioral health crisis • Migrant youth
- Community settings • Institutional environments • Systems of care

KEY POINTS

- Disparity in engagement of migrant youth in outpatient mental health care is noted, and emergency intervention is a frequent path of entry into mental health treatment.
- Adversities before, during, and after migration have impacts on youth psychological adjustment, and availability of parents, family, and other resources have mitigating effects and improve resilience.
- Suicidal ideation and behaviors are more frequent among some migrant youth compared with nonmigrant youth, and mental health challenges seen among migrant youth include post-traumatic stress disorder, depression, anxiety, and disruptive behaviors.
- Safety planning involves an at-risk youth but also engages family, caregivers, and possibly other supportive people to be an effective intervention against suicidality.
- Several brief interventions using psychoeducation and behavioral methods can be provided during an emergency interaction.
- Language and culture are not attended to sufficiently with migrant families when providing mental health care; disparities exist even with available resources.

INTRODUCTION

Some 43.3 million children in the world lived outside their native countries due to displacement by year's end in 2022.[1] War and political violence are major drivers of forced displacements.[2,3] Climate change-induced extreme weather has caused loss of homes, experiences of famine, and increased risks of worsening conflict around

[a] Department of Psychiatry and Behavioral Sciences, Montefiore Health Systems/ Albert Einstein College of Medicine, Bronx, NY, USA; [b] Department of Pediatrics, Montefiore Health Systems/ Albert Einstein College of Medicine, Bronx, NY, USA
* 1349 Lexington Avenue, #1EB, New York, NY 10128.
E-mail address: chocolatebirdie@live.com

Child Adolesc Psychiatric Clin N Am 33 (2024) 219–236
https://doi.org/10.1016/j.chc.2023.10.002

the world.[4–6] Although a large majority of children, adolescents, and their families are resilient when facing displacement and future circumstances, some will experience serious mental health challenges to the point of crisis. Migrant youth and families in crisis may present in hospital emergency rooms, in detention centers, at refugee camps, schools, community-based organizations, foster care agencies, or in the homes of relatives or other adults. Literature has shown refugee and other immigrant youth presenting to emergency rooms for their first mental health contact more often than non-refugee youth,[7] and disparities were seen in a European study of outpatient mental health care use among migrants compared with natives.[8–10] The encounter between mental health professionals and these youth during a psychiatric emergency may be a turning point to access treatment and other potential resources they would not have otherwise obtained on their own.

DEFINITIONS

Displacements affect youth (children and adolescents, collectively herein will be referred to as "youth(s)" in this article) who are migrants, asylum seekers, and refugees. The United Nations distinguishes the terms, "migrant" and "refugee" as follows: migrants "choose to move not because of a direct threat of persecution or death, but mainly to improve their lives by finding work, or in some cases for education, family reunion, or other reasons."[11] These other reasons may include loss of livelihood or available food due to climate change. Refugees are "persons fleeing armed conflict or persecution."[11] Amnesty International defines an "asylum seeker" as: a "person who has left their country and is seeking protection from persecution and serious human rights violations in another country, but who hasn't yet been legally recognized as a refugee."[12] This article will use the terms "migrants" and "refugees," and they will be used interchangeably as issues of legal status or reasons for migration will not be highlighted here. Of note, migrant youth, in many cases, are not free to choose to move, but rather are part of family or parental decision-making; minors themselves may not be emigrating by "choice." Importantly, regardless of status or terms, youth who are apart from their places of origin share common experiences that may lead to psychiatric emergencies; the considerations and approaches needed to care for these youth, whereas in emotional and behavioral crisis are similar.

The terms "emergency" and "crisis" and "urgent problems" have different interpretations, as per the American Psychiatric Association (APA) Report and Recommendations on Psychiatric Emergency and Crisis Services.[13] The APA report distinguishes between emergencies and urgent problems. An emergency is "a set of circumstances in which (1) the behavior or condition of an individual is perceived by someone......as having the potential to rapidly eventuate in a catastrophic outcome and (2) the resources available to understand and deal with the situation are not available at the time and place of the occurrence." Urgent problems are disturbances "where the situation is evolving more slowly, the feared outcome is not imminent, and attention can be delayed for a short time."[13] A "crisis" is an individually defined event (a true emergency or something less acute), whereas crisis services are a "continuum of alternative psychiatric emergency services.... intended to be available to the entire community" to avert hospitalization using the least restrictive means.[13,14] Clinicians will agree that most psychiatric issues characterized as "emergencies" are in fact, urgent problems, as they have often de-escalated by the time professional help is available, or interpreted to be more acute by caregivers than they actually are. Reasons for de-escalation of emergencies may include separation or removal from the precipitating environment or event and/or arrival of uniformed emergency personnel deterring further dangerous conduct. An example of crisis interpreted as emergency: a teacher learns that a calm teenager at school engaged in self-harm days before but sends them immediately to an emergency room. This article will use the terms emergency, crisis, and urgent problems interchangeably based on the community's lack of distinctions; the need for clinicians to intervene regardless of terms is the same.

BACKGROUND

Migrant youth face many hardships throughout migration. These include fleeing unsafe, impoverished, and/or oppressive countries. They may have witnessed or experienced horrific atrocities. Receiving communities may be unwelcoming, callous, and xenophobic. Acculturation and adjustment challenges to a new country may include language barriers, risk of deportation, social isolation, significant educational gaps, and/or economic stress. Despite the hardships, opportunities also abound. These include improved chances for learning, health care, employment, freedom of expression, and freedom from sociopolitical violence. Given the harms and gains faced by migrant youth, their ability to weather and adjust to the challenges ahead depends on several factors, namely, the types, extent, and number of harms experienced before and during migration, the youth's own constitution, the caregivers' ability to tolerate harms and their availability to their children, and finally, the postmigration circumstances.

CONSEQUENCES OF THE PANDEMIC AND OTHER DEVELOPMENTS

The coronavirus 2019 (COVID-19) pandemic incurred devastating social, emotional, and educational consequences for youth throughout the world and further decline in well-being above prior downward trends. More than 8 million children around the world were orphaned by COVID-19,[15] and learning poverty and large-scale learning loss among youth increased.[16,17] Depression and anxiety symptoms doubled among youth worldwide,[18] and emergency room presentations for self-harm in girls increased compared with pre-pandemic times.[19] In the United States, emergency room visits for adolescent girls suspected of suicide attempt increased by 51% in 2021,[20] and drug overdoses in youth increased by 109% between 2019 and 2021, and 41% of whom had prior mental health disorders.[21]

   In this current climate of worsening youth mental health, compounded by COVID-19, migrant youth have additional vulnerabilities. First, they often have had limited or no health care before their arrival to the host country; therefore, they are unlikely to have been screened for or identified with mental health problems. Second, stigma and cultural taboos may have barred identification and treatment for mental health conditions. Third, absent or deferred mental health care may cause advancement of mental health problems. Fourth, the biopsychosocial challenges, especially traumatic ones, of pre-, peri-, and postmigration may further challenge mental health. Finally, developmentally normal features of youth, such as immature emotional regulation, impulsivity, and poor judgment, faced with adversities of the migration process, may also result in crisis.

WHERE ARE THE EMERGENCIES?

Commonly, behavioral emergencies among migrant and refugee youth first present to hospital emergency rooms, rather than in outpatient environments.[7] A chart review of Austrian psychiatric emergency services showed that migrant youth used these services more than their native counterparts.[8] Other institutional settings where migrant and refugee youth may present in crisis include detention centers. Most of the psychiatric emergencies, however, originate in the community—at homes, classrooms, organizations such as foster care agencies, and shelters/temporary housing. As noted, acute symptoms may have diffused by the time a mental health assessment occurs. A crisis evaluation itself, though, provides opportunity for future care.

MENTAL HEALTH ISSUES IN MIGRANT YOUTH: TYPES OF BEHAVIORAL EMERGENCIES

Unaccompanied minor refugees (UMRs) have a high prevalence of depression, anxiety, post-traumatic stress disorder (PTSD), and behavioral problems.[22,23] A recent systematic review of 23 studies of UMR in European countries published between late 2017 and early 2022 found the prevalence of these mental health conditions ranging as follows: depression from 2.9% to 61.6%, anxiety from 32.6% to 38.2%, PTSD from 4.6% to 43%, and behavioral problems from 4% to 14.3%.[22] Therefore, it hardly, a surprise that some of these problems present as psychiatric emergencies, which may include: acutely suicidal/self-injurious behavior, severely disruptive or aggressive behavior, prolonged and extreme dysregulation of affect, severe anxiety, psychosis, behaviors due to drug or alcohol intoxication, reactions to trauma, and acute mental status changes due to organic causes such as medical conditions, substance intoxication, or withdrawal.[24] This article addresses two very common types of emergency affecting migrant youth: suicidal behaviors and agitation. Special attention will be given to matters of language, safety planning, culture, and impacts of the migrant experiences on childhood development and general mental health.

As with nonmigrant populations, most migrant youth with mental health problems forgo diagnosis and treatment. Engagement of refugee populations in outpatient mental health care remains low as compared with emergency room care, attributed often to cultural and language barriers, stigma, and poor clinician understanding of this population's needs.[25]

Determinants of migrant youth's psychological adjustment to a new life include an individual's constitution, developmental stage, and flexibility to adapt to changes. Additional determinants include duration, intensity, and frequency of exposures to traumatic stress, prior and ongoing caregiving, family and social supports, resources such as stable housing, food, material goods, and availability of school and larger community.[26] A thorough evaluation of these factors is necessary along with usual history and examination following a psychiatric crisis. Once protective factors such as peer/family, social, and religious supports are identified, incorporating these elements into recommendations for future care is imperative.

GENERAL APPROACH TO PSYCHIATRIC EMERGENCIES

Managing any psychiatric emergency requires an order of operations (no matter who is affected or where it occurs) as follows: *triage* to identify the level of danger, *establish safety* and readiness for safety planning (including transport if necessary for higher level of care), *enable communication*, *engage caregivers* and immediate family or social network, *provide* appropriate *brief interventions*, and *connect* to further resources. A full psychiatric evaluation occurs in tandem with these tasks.

TRIAGE AND SAFETY

The level of risk must be established to know if it is safe to proceed with a psychiatric evaluation in the absence of life-saving support, monitoring, or other emergency interventions. The highest risk cases where life is in immediate danger (eg, overdose, life-threatening suicide attempt) would require involvement with emergency personnel and transport to a hospital, emergency room, or other location where life-saving measures are provided. The telephone triage tool, the Mental Health Triage Scale (MHTS) (www.ukmentalhealthtriagescale.org),[27,28] provides a useful framework for recognizing and managing risks. Other risk categories are described by the MHTS as follows: very high risk (eg, actively suicidal, aggressive, showing signs of abnormal mental status or unpredictable behavior), high risk (eg, suicidal ideation [SI] without plan, impulsive), moderate risk (eg, significantly distressed, socially isolated, or significant risk factors), or low risk, nonurgent presentations, which permit deferred mental health care in an outpatient setting (eg, depressed in primary care).[27]

Very high-risk presentations in youth may warrant further care in an institutional environment such as an emergency room or hospital, although a highly equipped mobile crisis service may be able to provide stepped-down care.[29] Hospital-level care is needed especially if the cause of the disturbance is not known and may be a threat to health such as cases of delirium, where laboratory tests, imaging, monitoring, and treatments with medications such as antibiotics and neuroleptics can take place. In the case of violent youth, in the absence of personnel trained in safe de-escalation and/or application of restraints, urgent transport to a setting with qualified staff (in appropriate numbers) will be needed. In addition, very high-risk patients may require safety interventions such as 1:1 supervision, placement in a secured space free of dangerous items, and assessment for level of acuity of the psychiatric presentation. These levels of acuity, usually in cases of agitation, would be classified into mild, moderate, or severe. A mild level of acuity can be managed using non-pharmacologic, de-escalating behavioral strategies (eg, calming techniques, reduction of stimuli, offering food, or comfort items). A traumatized youth who is responding to a triggering situation with agitation and possibly dissociation may especially benefit from reduction of environmental stimuli and grounding techniques. A moderate level of acuity would likely warrant more advanced behavioral techniques or the use of emergency medications by mouth to alleviate symptoms, whereas severe level would require containment using seclusion and restraint and/or emergency medications for sedation given by mouth or injection.[30]

High-risk patients generally warrant urgent attention either through a mobile crisis team or other outreach worker may be managed in the community or may need further referral for a higher level of care, depending on the ability to safety plan, arrange for close follow-up, and availability of supports and protective factors.[27]

Moderate-risk patients who pose no immediate danger to self or others warrant attention that may be deferred briefly (hours to days) and are appropriate for assessment at the community level. Finally, low- or minimal-risk patients on triage may be deferred for assessment on a nonurgent basis, usually via outpatient mental health referral, or through lower levels of support such as primary care, or with information/advice only.[28,31]

Discussion of Case 1

Suicide safety

Suicide has become a major public health issue, as the fourth leading cause of death worldwide in 15- to 29-year-olds, and in the United States, the second and third leading cause of death in 10- to 14-year-olds and 15- to 24-year-olds, respectively[32](Box 1). Migrant youth surveys from various settings and sources (eg, schools, national registries, clinics, labor, and detention camps) show that they have higher rates of self-harm and suicide attempts compared with nonmigrants, and that migration itself can be a risk factor for non-suicidal self-injury and suicide attempts.[33–35]

Box 1
Discussion of case 1

Case 1: Suicidality

Leela is a 16-year-old young woman brought to the attention of a consulting psychiatrist by a peer because she was experiencing suicidal ideation with plan to take an overdose of pre-scribed medications. She was evacuated from Afghanistan 2 months before the assessment, just after the country's takeover by the Taliban, currently residing in temporary housing with acquaintances and an adult cousin at a military compound in the United States on temporary humanitarian parole. Four months before the evaluation, she survived a bombing at her school after weeks of threat and demands to shut down. Leela also belonged to a persecuted minority group, the Hazera. Although she sustained only minor injuries, she witnessed the killing of many girls, including several close friends, and saw considerable blood and gore at the scene of the attack. Almost immediately and since the event, she has been sleepless, without appe-tite, reexperiencing the bombing while awake, and suffering nightmares when asleep. She has constant low mood, guilt for having survived, intermittent suicidal ideation, yearning for her parents, and hopelessness about the future. Three weeks before this assessment, she received health screening and was identified by a mental health practitioner as having depres-sion and post-traumatic stress disorder (PTSD). She was then prescribed an antidepressant, fluoxetine, and scheduled for biweekly follow-up appointments at the clinic. Neither individ-ual psychotherapy nor any formal school arrangements were yet available at the facility, so Leela only received non-governmental organization (NGO) run recreational programming. As for her medication, it was kept among her belongings, and she oversaw dispensing her own pills. She admitted to forgetting about the medicine and missed several doses over the last week. None of the women in her living space were aware that she was on medication, nor did she speak to anyone about her distress until her friend noticed that she was more with-drawn and had stopped eating meals with her. She admitted to her friend how she was feeling, which led the friend to take her to the medical clinic, to receive the attention of a consulting psychiatrist. On evaluation, she was found to be of expected age, neatly dressed in a mix of Asian and Western attire, detached and affectively flat appearing, but cooperative with normal speech and a fair command of understandable English. Her suicidal ideation was inter-mittent, but absent at the time of interview, nor did she endorse any hallucinations or delu-sions, and had fair to good insight and judgment, good impulse control, and cognition that was age appropriate.

Clinical Questions
1. How can Leela's risks for suicide be identified and addressed?
2. How can suicide safety planning be carried out effectively in this community, especially with cultural, language, and housing barriers?
3. What are other prior adverse and traumatic events that need to be considered in evaluation and treatment planning for Leela?
4. How can medication administration, monitoring, and response be improved here?
5. Are there any brief interventions that may be helpful in Leela's case?

European chart reviews of outpatient emergency services and psychiatric inpatient admissions show migrant youth have higher numbers of suicide attempts compared with nonmigrant youth.[8] In addition, migrant youth have higher rates of PTSD, disrup-tive behavior, conduct disorders, impulse control disorders, and personality disorders compared with native youth at inpatient psychiatric discharge in an Italian study.[35] Among war exposed youth, daily stressors (economic/housing/food, interpersonal conflicts, and so forth) play a significant role in psychological adjustment.[23] Still, with a wide range of cultural differences in response to the immigration experience noted in the literature, it is difficult to generalize any one group's mental health expe-riences without taking sociopolitical circumstances, culture, individual and family risk, and protective factors into account.

For many cultures, the topic of suicide remains stigmatized,[25,35] and conversations with youth, caregivers, and families on suicide prevention may be difficult to initiate. However, experts consider open and supportive conversations around mental health and suicide as protective and mitigating against suicide and therefore imperative for clinicians to engage all patients and family in these dialogues.[36] Further, the availability and use of linguistically and culturally informed suicide prevention resources such as translated public educational materials for patients and families, crisis hotlines in appropriate languages, and family communication training has been demonstrated to be helpful in reducing and protecting against suicidal behaviors in youth.[37–39] In Case 1, Leela must be apprised of the need to involve her cousin/guardian and possibly friend in managing SI and behavior in the community, as lack of parental/family and other social supports elevate her risks for suicide, whereas the presence of these supports are protective and may reduce suicidal behavior.[39–41]

Can Leela engage in safety planning, perhaps with the help of her cousin and friend? Given her risks for suicide, which include prior SI, stressful life events, and diagnosed psychiatric disorders of depression and PTSD, suicide screening is imperative. Screening tools such as Ask Suicide Questions or the Columbia Suicide Severity Rating Scale might be used, and further risk assessment using a tool such as the Suicide Assessment Five-Step Evaluation and Triage or the Brief Suicide Safety Assessment is indicated.[42–44] If screening and risk assessment determine a moderate or high risk for suicide, a comprehensive clinical evaluation is required. If screening, assessment, and clinical evaluation deem that outpatient management is safe, then the clinician, youth, and those providing support (eg, caregiver, friend) can develop a suicide safety plan together. Safety planning is an evidence-based strategy to reduce the risk of suicide.[45] A review of adult studies shows safety planning to be associated with improvements across several domains: reduction in SI and behaviors, reduction in mental health symptoms, fewer hospitalizations, and better treatment engagement.[46–48] In youth, the evidence for safety planning is emergent but promising.[49] The standard safety plan is a written document generated by a clinician and patient (in this case, youth), with involvement of other people in the patient's life. Basic literacy in at least one native language is helpful (but not required) as the plan is usually written (even if simply worded). However, groups with low written literacy rates such as refugees have had positive results with safety planning using alternate methods such as images, drawings, and pictures.[50] Further, migrant youth may be fluent or proficient in more than one spoken language, which can expand options to develop a safety plan. Limitations on safety planning are noted, however, including low availability of templates in languages other than English (LOE) and Spanish, and few studies providing evidence for their use and validity across non-English speaking groups and younger populations; nonetheless, accurate translation and cultural adaptation of a completed safety plan is recommended.

Several types of safety plan are available, including the well-known, Stanley and Brown Safety Intervention.[45] The first part of a safety plan identifies and lists the individual's warning signs/triggers for SI (eg, change of mood, racing negative thoughts, pacing, and poor sleep). The next part generates a list coping behaviors that could counteract dangerous urges or thoughts (eg, drawing, taking a walk, and breathing exercise). The third part limits the youth's access to violent means by removing or securing dangerous items (firearms, sharps, medications, chemicals, and ropes). Additional resources to include in the plan are suicide or crisis hotlines/helplines for call or text and locations/contacts of emergency rooms and hospitals. Finally, contact information for friends, family, teachers, or familiar health/mental health professionals to be used during a crisis is listed. Some safety plans also list reasons to live. Safety plans are available through smartphone apps, on the Internet, or in print form.[51–53]

Although experts (the American Academy of Pediatrics, American Psychological Association, American Academy of Family Medicine, Royal College of Psychiatrists)[54–57] recommend safety planning (also known as crisis planning) to mitigate risk around future suicidal behavior, concern has been raised that a poorly executed suicide safety plan (done in rushed, emergency situation) without adequate engagement of the patient(s) or members of their support group in preparing it may be unhelpful in preventing future self-harm.[58] For a plan to be successful, experts recommend a high level of engagement from the patient, social support members, and clinician in coproducing the safety plan.[58]

Restriction of access to lethal means in an immediate living environment, whether in a home or a facility, can be challenging; access to personal spaces may not be granted to a clinician. Only where child protective services or home visiting programs (eg, visiting nurse, home-based crisis intervention program) are involved, are additional supports available to help youth and families secure their environment. However, with the caregiver and youth's permission, telehealth may allow clinicians more involvement in this task, including visualization of living spaces. Case 1 involves a military base, which has institutional features (structures, services, and security), but it may also have aspects that are difficult to control, as in the general community. For example, unsafe, covert behaviors of individuals in communal living spaces are unlikely to be monitored and therefore risky. Adult supervised medication storage would be an intervention on the safety plan. Finally, if Leela cannot be engaged in safety planning with clinician and family member involvement, she may need observation and care in a more secure environment such as an emergency room or psychiatric inpatient unit for further treatment.

Family separation

Does Leela have any contact with immediate family while overseas? Disruption of the family unit and parent–child relationship(s) is undoubtedly one of the most adverse events that could happen. Parent–child separation, even if brief (days to months), can be associated with increased mental health problems in immigrant children even after reunification.[59,60] This was observed in a cross-sectional survey of 425 children ages 4–17 year and their mothers in detention at the US Mexican Border in 2018. All of the children in the study had higher than normal rates of emotional problems, peer problems, and total difficulties on the Strengths and Difficulties Questionnaire (SDQ). Of these children, 17% had been separated from parents before reunification. Scores on the SDQ for the previously separated children showed higher rates of emotional problems compared with non-separated children (49% vs 29%, respectively) and higher rates of total difficulties (15% vs 9%, respectively).[59] Furthermore, previously separated children's SDQ scores were similarly high regardless of the length of separation (shorter vs longer duration).[59] Disconnect from her parents and siblings may be adding to Leela's despondency and anxiety. Although contact with family is of value (barring a contentious relationship between the youth and family), awareness of ongoing danger faced by family back home and uncertainty around their well-being may further cause anxiety. Supportive adults substituting for parents have an important role to play in the well-being of children and teens. Family-centered interventions are preferred in many cultures and may provide greater yield than those that are only individually focused. In addition, folk, religious, and spiritual healing have significant roles across cultures, and inquiry around availability of such supports is appropriate and potentially helpful.[61] In this particular case, consultation with an imam or other religious leader, if available, may provide insights and trusted access to mental health dialogues in this community.

Other prior adversities and traumas

As a young woman and ethnic minority, Leela has been subjected to multiple severe toxic stressors resulting from long-standing discrimination, oppression, and harassment. A population-based study of Afghan women (ages 15–80 years) revealed that the prevalence of major depression and SI was extremely high among women from Taliban-controlled areas (73%–78% for depression and 28% for SI), compared with women in non-Taliban-controlled areas (28% and 18%, respectively).[62] Because Leela's country had been a conflict zone for four decades, she and her family lived in a climate of danger, unpredictability, and constant hardship. A general population survey (ages 15+) of a war-impacted Afghan province showed exposure to higher numbers of traumatic events to be associated with a high prevalence of depressive and post-traumatic stress symptoms.[63] A school-based survey of Afghan children between 11 and 16 and their caregivers also found that exposures to multiple traumatic events were predictors of poor mental health in children and caregivers.[64] Finally, an epidemiologic study in a war-torn, Arab country found that exposure to war increased the risk of first-onset anxiety (eg, social anxiety disorder, PTSD, generalized anxiety disorder), mood (major depression and dysthymia), and impulse control disorders.[65] Hence, inquiry around hostilities faced at home before evacuation, including the types and level of exposure to war traumata along with parental/caregiver mental health, will clarify risks and guide treatment planning.

Language barrier

Leela, her cousin, and friend should have an interpreter (Dari or Pashto, depending on preference) for this interview. Despite appearance of English proficiency, improved clinical care is more likely with professional interpretation.[66] Informal translation through family members or acquaintances is all too common, has the potential for inaccuracies, and may disregard patient privacy. Disparities due to language barrier during pediatric emergency care have been described[67,68]; even when language needs are considered in clinical settings, the care received by these groups continues to fall short. Pediatric inpatient and emergency room research on interactions between health care providers and patients/families who speak LOE shows that despite availability of interpreter services, communication inequities still occur. Examples include under-use of interpreters and/or lower engagement with (LOE) patient families in ongoing care (eg, less inclusion of such families during inpatient round discussions or provision of treatment updates after rounds).[69,70] A call exists for greater representation of multilingual patients and families in pediatric research, as studies generally exclude these groups[71,72]; a review of original pediatric research published between 2012 and 2021 showed evidence that non-English speaking communities were underrepresented.[72] It is also not in Leela's best interest to bypass an interpreter, given the connection with first language and emotions, and the fact that she has only been in the United States for 2 months (older adolescents may be disadvantaged because they acquire second language proficiency at a slower rate than school-aged children).[73]

Medication monitoring and compliance

Case 1 shows an oversight in the US Federal Drug Agency (FDA) boxed warning recommendation for patient monitoring for the first few weeks of starting a selective serotonin reuptake inhibitor (SSRI) in younger patients (see **Box 1**). Adult clinicians may forget the recommendation for weekly then biweekly check-ins for the first 2 months of therapy to monitor for suicidality in youth ≤ 24 years of age. Initial studies on suicidality among youth led to the boxed warning on SSRIs for people less than 25 year.[74] Although evidence is lacking for the FDA monitoring schedule, the prescribing clinician may consider compliance with local, professional safety standards.

As for the undercompliance with taking medication, a written chart/log or smartphone app reminder to keep track of doses may help. A pill box with days of the week labeled might also be helpful. Psychoeducation on the number of weeks needed for response to an SSRI is paramount, as patients commonly stop antidepressants prematurely. Appreciating cultural stigma for medication treatment and sensitivity for cultural beliefs and family expectations around medications (eg, 1 or a few doses will not result in a "cure") is necessary. In Leela's case, was her aunt uninformed of ongoing medication therapy because the teenager was embarrassed about the treatment for her problem? Was there a misunderstanding due to language or other reasons around how the medication was to be taken? Was there hesitancy or distrust around recommendations from health care providers of a different cultural background? Do they believe the cause of illness was amenable to treatment with medications, and what is their culturally specific expectation around recovery?[61] Further, building a caregiver–family alliance may help increase trust and motivation to follow through on treatment recommendations.

Some additional concerns must be mentioned with regard to the use and availability of medications in settings such as a refugee camp. Disruptions in medication supply or lack of access to medications may occur in the case of inadequate security at the camp, especially if looting of goods such as food, medications, and other materials is experienced with any regularity.[75] In addition, if the medications are not free of charge, refugees have cited cost as a barrier to obtaining medications, more so than their community counterparts. An additional barrier to obtaining prescribed medication includes inadequate supply at local or institutional pharmacies, as noted in a survey of Syrian refugees residing in Lebanon.[76] Therefore, the decision to initiate pharmacotherapy in youth, must be judiciously made, and often deferred, given the uncertainties around maintaining access to medications under these circumstances.

Brief interventions
Emergency circumstances lend themselves only to brief psychiatric interventions. Importantly, most of such interventions for children and youth are non-pharmacologic. Many such interventions exist: psychoeducation, safety planning, behavioral activation through activity scheduling, relaxation training, brief cognitive behavioral exercises, sleep hygiene education, parent training, and motivational interviewing. Behavioral activation may be especially useful in Leela's case as it has been shown to improve depressive symptoms and functioning in adolescents as well as adults,[77] and activity scheduling is an exercise easily initiated during a brief contact. Sleep hygiene education is another brief intervention, given that poor sleep is a predictor of SI and attempts, and improvements in sleep may reduce the risks of future suicidal behaviors.[38,78] Brief parent intervention includes psychoeducation around communication. Outpatient interventions include parent training, parental support, and strategies promoting parental empowerment and self-efficacy through community engagement and network building. Such interventions have shown promise in improving socioemotional and developmental health in children and families.[79]

Discussion of Case 2

Placement and development
Language development is essential in children's future emotional, social, and academic achievement[80](**Box 2**). In Case 2, it is likely that language immaturity contributes to Omar and Abdel's disruptive behaviors, but there are some other challenges

---

Box 2
Discussion of case 1

Case 2: Agitation

Omar and Luis, ages 4 and 6 year, are brothers in foster care, brought to the urgent attention of a consulting psychiatrist at the agency for extremely disruptive and aggressive behavior in the home. The boys were returned to the agency by the foster parent who did not welcome them back. Early history is unknown, but the boys are unaccompanied minors, separated from their parents before entering the country. It was discovered that the children were smuggled in with unrelated adults through Central America and subject to repeated abuse. After they were apprehended by immigration, the adults were deported, the boys were taken into federal custody and placed in long-term foster care. They are believed to be Guatemalan and have been in the United States for 4 months. The whereabouts of the parents are unknown. They understand and speak Spanish, although Omar does not use full sentences. Luis has been learning English through children's television programs. Although Omar has learned some words, he has inadequate vocabulary for age in either language. They were placed with an English-speaking family for 2 months where communication at home was limited, and they were not enrolled in school. Examination reveals them both to be overly friendly with the examiner and eager to play with toys, although in a frenetic and disorganized manner—moving from item to item without completing any actions, breaking building blocks into pieces as soon as a structure is made, all while making very loud sounds. Omar plays alone but Luis is often intruding on his space and instigating a fight whenever interactions occur, but when supervised, they can behave safely and play less aggressively.

Clinical Questions
1. Therapeutic interventions may help with disruptive behaviors in such young children?
2. Did the foster placement for the boys impact their language development and contribute to intermittent aggressive behaviors?
3. What parenting interventions would be helpful to support foster parents to have a more successful placement?
4. What therapeutic interventions may help with disruptive behaviors in such young children?

(see **Box 2**). Unfortunately, multiple disrupted foster placements are common among both domestic and unaccompanied minors in foster care.[81] In addition, placement in homes where the language and culture of foster parents and child(ren) are unmatched is also common, despite recommendation that a foster family shares the same language and culture with the child(ren), allowing for better adjustment and development.[82,83] In the case of the boys' English learning (especially for Omar, the preschooler), it may be slow to progress as demonstrated in a longitudinal study of children and language acquisition. The study showed that mastery of a first language in the earlier years was predictive of competence in learning subsequent languages. At least 4 to 5 years or more of learning predicted competency in a second language.[73,83] In the case of both boys, development of their native Spanish was likely inhibited in the home where they were placed. However, language barrier aside, a caring home itself may still help with other aspects of language learning; in a study of maltreated children, placement in nurturing foster care benefited receptive early language development more than placement with (maltreating) birth parents.[80]

Traumatic play
Disorganized, repetitive, and aggressive play is typical of young children who have experienced trauma and represents reenactments of traumatic events. The connection between certain play, behaviors, and triggers resulting in post-traumatic reactions

is not always apparent, nor can very young children make verbal connections to events that were stressful.[84] Foster families may be uninformed about children's past exposures and experiences, even when trained for "therapeutic foster care." They may further benefit from psychoeducation on the meaning of aggressive play, and how best to safely facilitate, rather than interrupt or extinguish it. Recognition that poor emotional regulation is a result of trauma, and that play is a vehicle for children's expression of traumatic experiences, rather than purposeful misbehavior, is important parental education. Parental understanding of the children's behaviors is necessary to permit empathic reactions and prevent punitive caregiver responses.[85] In addition, orienting parents to the "3 pillars of trauma-informed care" is helpful—establishing safety for children, making connections through stable relationships between caregiving adults and children, and helping children manage emotions.[85]

Educational concerns

Aggressive assessment for special education and services such as speech therapy is indicated in at least one of these boys with probable speech delay, and classification may benefit the other boy through smaller class placement, given difficulties functioning without high levels of structure and supervision. Obtaining services for immigrant children with developmental delays has been shown to be difficult.[86] Correct educational placement is also essential as the boys have already had a subpar experience with foster placement and need not experience it again in their education. The agency must be apprised of evaluation and placement needs as ignoring them may lead to worsening of disruptive behaviors.

Interventions

Emergency pharmacotherapy with these boys is contraindicated given response to behavioral methods such as verbal redirection, distraction, and structuring of activities. The first-line approach to de-escalation of agitated patients favors verbal and nonverbal methods over more restrictive approaches such as chemical or physical restraints.[87,88] However, referral for future pharmacologic treatments may be necessary once outpatient diagnostic assessment and behavioral interventions (eg, parent management training, psychotherapies using play) have been initiated, if disruptive behaviors persist. Such assessment and interventions would not generally take place in crisis or emergency circumstances. Single-session parenting interventions that are achievable during a crisis interaction include providing psychoeducation, teaching active listening, and helping label difficult emotions.[89,90] Parenting interventions in general, including those targeting refugees and other displaced families, are usually provided over multiple sessions, often in group format, involve positive parenting and family communication methods, and usually delivered through community-based programs.[91]

SUMMARY

Migrant youth mental health needs are first often addressed when in crisis and not through outpatient care. This is due to various reasons, including stigma or advancement of problems to higher acuity, but also due to limited engagement of culturally and linguistically appropriate resources promoting mental health literacy, and limited understanding by clinicians on best care for this population. Evaluation and care for psychiatric emergencies are not limited to immediate circumstances but are on a continuum of mental health care, requiring a multimodal approach with several systems of care integrating family and community resources. Successful disposition planning including these elements may help avert the next crisis.

CLINICS CARE POINTS

- Migrant youth are likely to present for mental health intervention under emergency circumstances rather than in outpatient clinics.

- As with nonmigrant youth, triage around level of dangerousness and appropriateness to safely manage psychiatric crisis in the community must be done, and referral to emergency rooms or inpatient units for safety may be indicated.

- De-escalation of agitation using behavioral techniques is preferred over pharmacologic management of agitation and disruptive behaviors, especially in younger children.

- Safety planning is an evidence-based intervention found in adult studies to reduce SI and behaviors, reduce negative mental health symptoms, improve treatment engagement, and lead to fewer hospitalizations. The evidence for safety planning in youth is emergent but promising as well.

- An effective safety plan is a cocreated document that involves the youth, mental health clinician, and caregiver/family/social support members as participants.

- Community-level management is preferred over institutional care using resources drawing from various systems (community-based organizations, mobile crisis teams, crisis hotlines, and so forth) if youth and family can participate in safety planning.

- Several brief interventions are possible under emergency circumstances, which include safety planning, psychoeducation, behavioral activation, teaching active listening and labeling of emotions, and sleep hygiene.

- Professional interpreters, translated psychoeducational materials, and cultural liaison/advocates for migrant families are not used often enough even if available, but they improve care and may improve future engagement in mental health treatment.

- Youth separated from parents experience more distress and emotional difficulties than youth who migrate with their parents/caregivers.

- Foster placements of unaccompanied minors should be matched whenever possible for language and culture with foster families.

- Appropriate early development of a first language facilitates second language development; incomplete early language development in a native language makes acquisition of a second language more difficult.

- Migrant youth with developmental concerns are at risk for being overlooked for necessary educational services; inadequate assessment and incorrect educational placement of such youth can lead to worsening of disruptive behaviors.

DISCLOSURE

The author has nothing to disclose.

REFERENCES

1. Number of displaced children reaches new high of 43.3 million (unicef.org) Accessed September 4, 2023.
2. Boothby N. Political violence and development: an ecologic approach to children in war zones. Child Adolesc Psychiatr Clin N Am 2008;17(3):497–vii.
3. Joshi PT, Fayyad JA. Displaced children: the psychological implications. Child Adolesc Psychiatr Clin N Am 2015;24(4):715–30.
4. Climate | National Oceanic and Atmospheric Administration (noaa.gov) Accessed May 31, 2023.

5. Mach KJ, Kraan CM, Adger WN, et al. Climate as a risk factor for armed conflict. Nature 2019;571(7764):193–7.

6. 4487_002_When Rain Turns to Dust: Understanding and Responding to the Combined Impact of Armed Conflicts and the Climate and Environment Crisis on people's lives; 07.2020; PDF (icrc.org) Accessed May 31, 2023.

7. Saunders NR, Gill PJ, Holder L, et al. Use of the emergency department as a first point of contact for mental health care by immigrant youth in Canada: a population-based study. CMAJ (Can Med Assoc J) 2018;190(40):E1183–91.

8. Akkaya-Kalayci T, Popow C, Waldhör T, et al. Psychiatric emergencies of minors with and without migration background. Psychiatrische Akutvorstellungen von Minderjährigen mit und ohne Migrationshintergrund. Neuropsychiatry 2017; 31(1):1–7.

9. Koopmans GT, Uiters E, Devillé W, et al. The use of outpatient mental health care services of migrants vis-a-vis Dutch natives: equal access? Int J Soc Psychiatr 2013;59(4):342–50.

10. Kieseppä V, Torniainen-Holm M, Jokela M, et al. Immigrants' mental health service use compared to that of native Finns: a register study. Soc Psychiatr Psychiatr Epidemiol 2020;55(4):487–96.

11. Refugee vs. migrant: Which is right and why it matters (unrefugees.org) Published 2015. Accessed May 31, 2023.

12. Refugees, Asylum Seekers and Migrants - Amnesty International Published 2023. Accessed May 31, 2023.

13. Microsoft Word - Emergency Services Final - Use This One.doc (psychiatry.org) APA Task Force on Emergency Services, Report and Recommendations Regarding Psychiatric Emergency and Crisis Services. Published 2002. Accessed May 31, 2023.

14. Janssens A, Hayen S, Walraven V, et al. Emergency psychiatric care for children and adolescents: a literature review. Pediatr Emerg Care 2013;29(9):1041–50.

15. covid19orphans-widget (imperialcollegelondon.github.io) Published December 31, 2022. Accessed May 31, 2023.

16. The pandemic has had devastating impacts on learning. What will it take to help students catch up? | Brookings Published March 3, 2022. Accessed May 31, 2023.

17. National Academies of Sciences, Engineering, and Medicine. Addressing the long-term effects of the COVID-19 pandemic on children and families. Washington, DC: The National Academies Press; 2023. https://doi.org/10.17226/26809. . Published 2023. Accessed May 31, 2023.

18. Racine N, McArthur BA, Cooke JE, et al. Global prevalence of depressive and anxiety symptoms in children and adolescents during COVID-19: a meta-analysis. JAMA Pediatr 2021;175(11):1142–50.

19. Wong BH, Cross S, Zavaleta-Ramírez P, et al. Self-harm in children and adolescents who presented at emergency units during the COVID-19 pandemic: an international retrospective cohort study [published online ahead of print, 2023 feb 16]. J Am Acad Child Adolesc Psychiatry 2023;S0890-8567(23):00062.

20. Yard E, Radhakrishnan L, Ballesteros MF, et al. Emergency department visits for suspected suicide attempts among persons aged 12-25 Years before and during the COVID-19 pandemic - United States, January 2019-May 2021. MMWR Morb Mortal Wkly Rep 2021;70(24):888–94. Published 2021 Jun 18.

21. Tanz LJ, Dinwiddie AT, Mattson CL, et al. Drug overdose deaths among persons aged 10-19 Years - United States, july 2019-december 2021. MMWR Morb Mortal Wkly Rep 2022;71(50):1576–82.

22. Daniel-Calveras A, Baldaquí N, Baeza I. Mental health of unaccompanied refugee minors in Europe: a systematic review. Child Abuse Negl 2022;133:105865.
23. Newnham EA, Pearson RM, Stein A, et al. Youth mental health after civil war: the importance of daily stressors. Br J Psychiatry 2015;206(2):116–21.
24. Barth SE. Psychiatric emergencies. Child Adolesc Psychiatr Clin N Am 2003;12(4).
25. Pumariega AJ, Rothe E. Cultural considerations in child and adolescent psychiatric emergencies and crises. Child Adolesc Psychiatr Clin N Am 2003;12(4):723–vii.
26. Guidance for Mental Health Screening during the Domestic Medical Examination for Newly Arrived Refugees | Immigrant and Refugee Health | CDC Published 2022. Accessed May 28, 2023.
27. Sands N, Elsom S, Colgate R. UK mental health triage scale guidelines. Wales: UK Mental Health Triage Scale Project; 2015.
28. Sands N, Elsom S, Colgate R, et al. Development and interrater reliability of the UK mental health triage scale. Int J Ment Health Nurs 2016;25(4):330–6.
29. Fylla I, Fousfouka E, Kostoula M, et al. The interventions of a mobile mental health unit on the refugee crisis on a Greek island. Psych 2022;4:49–59.
30. Heyneman EK. The aggressive child. Child Adolesc Psychiatr Clin N Am 2003;12(4):667–vii.
31. Mental health of adolescents (who.int) Published 2021. Accessed May 31, 2023.
32. WISQARS Data Visualization (cdc.gov) Published 2022. Accessed May 31, 2023.
33. Plener PL, Munz LM, Allroggen M, et al. Immigration as risk factor for non-suicidal self-injury and suicide attempts in adolescents in Germany. Child Adolesc Psychiatry Ment Health 2015;9(34). https://doi.org/10.1186/s13034-015-0065-4.
34. Basu A, Boland A, Witt K, et al. Suicidal behaviour, including ideation and self-harm, in young migrants: a systematic review. Int J Environ Res Publ Health 2022;19(8329):1–17. https://doi.org/10.3390/ijerph19148329.
35. Loi E, Andriuolo G, LA Boria P, et al. Psychiatric emergencies in migrant adolescents. Minerva Pediatr 2022. https://doi.org/10.23736/S2724-5276.22.06635-6 [published online ahead of print, 2022 Feb 22].
36. Talk Away the Dark | AFSP Published 2023. Accessed May 31, 2023.
37. Aichberger MC, Heredia Montesinos A, Bromand Z, et al. Suicide attempt rates and intervention effects in women of Turkish origin in Berlin. Eur Psychiatr 2015;30(4):480–5.
38. Brent DA, McMakin DL, Kennard BD, et al. Protecting adolescents from self-harm: a critical review of intervention studies. J Am Acad Child Adolesc Psychiatry 2013;52(12):1260–71.
39. Özlü-Erkilic Z, Diehm R, Wenzel T, et al. Transcultural differences in suicide attempts among children and adolescents with and without migration background, a multicentre study: in Vienna, Berlin, Istanbul. Eur Child Adolesc Psychiatr 2022;31(11):1671–83.
40. Cho YB, Haslam N. Suicidal ideation and distress among immigrant adolescents: the role of acculturation, life stress, and social support. J Youth Adolesc 2010;39(4):370–9.
41. Boyd DT, Quinn CR, Jones KV, et al. Suicidal ideations and attempts within the family context: the role of parent support, bonding, and peer experiences with suicidal behaviors. J Racial Ethn Health Disparities 2022;9(5):1740–9.
42. About the Protocol The Columbia Lighthouse Project (The Columbia-Suicide Severity Rating Scale (C-SSRS)/The Columbia Protocol). Published 2016. Accessed May 31, 2023.

43. Evaluation and Triage card : Safe-T Card. (SMA) 09-4432. CMHS-NSP-0193. (samhsa.gov), Published 2009. Accessed May 31, 2023.
44. bssa_ed_youth_asq_nimh_toolkit.pdf (nih.gov), Published 2020. Accessed May 31, 2023.
45. Stanley B, Brown GK. Safety planning intervention: a brief intervention to mitigate suicide risk. Cognit Behav Pract 2012;19(2):256–64.
46. Weber AN, Michail M, Thompson A, et al. Psychiatric emergencies: assessing and managing suicidal ideation. Med Clin North Am 2017;101(3):553–71.
47. Ferguson M, Rhodes K, Loughhead M, et al. The effectiveness of the safety planning intervention for adults experiencing suicide-related distress: a systematic review. Arch Suicide Res 2022;26(3):1022–45.
48. Marshall CA, Crowley P, Carmichael D, et al. Effectiveness of suicide safety planning interventions: a systematic review informing occupational therapy. Can J Occup Ther 2023;90(2):208–36.
49. Abbott-Smith S, Ring N, Dougall N, et al. Suicide prevention: what does the evidence show for the effectiveness of safety planning for children and young people? - a systematic scoping review [published online ahead of print, 2023 Apr 13]. J Psychiatr Ment Health Nurs 2023. https://doi.org/10.1111/jpm.12928.
50. Ferguson M, Posselt M, McIntyre H, et al. Staff perspectives of safety planning as a suicide prevention intervention for people of refugee and asylum-seeker background [published correction appears in crisis. 2022. Crisis 2022;43(4):331–8.
51. Staying Safe (4 For Mental Health suicide educational website) Accessed May 31, 2023.
52. Home | My Safety Plan (create a personalized SP for individual with warning signs, coping methods, distractions, supports, creating a safer environment), Vibrant Emotional Health. Published 2021. Accessed May 31, 2023.
53. Suicide Safe Mobile App | SAMHSA Publications and Digital Products Published 2015. Accessed May 31, 2023.
54. Brief Interventions that Can Make a Difference in Suicide Prevention (aap.org) Updated February 22, 2023. Accessed May 31, 2023.
55. Mobile apps designed to help prevent suicide (apaservices.org) Published February, 2023. Accessed May 31, 2023.
56. Norris DR, Clark MS. The suicidal patient: evaluation and management. Am Fam Physician 2021;103(7):417–21.
57. college-report-cr229-self-harm-and-suicide.pdf (rcpsych.ac.uk) Published July, 2020. Accessed May 31, 2023.
58. House A. Self-harm and suicide in adults: will safety plans keep people safe after self-harm? BJPsych Bull 2022;46(1):1–3.
59. MacLean SA, Agyeman PO, Walther J, et al. Mental health of children held at a United States immigration detention center. Soc Sci Med 2019;230:303–8.
60. MacLean SA, Agyeman PO, Walther J, et al. Characterization of the mental health of immigrant children separated from their mothers at the U.S.-Mexico border. Psychiatr Res 2020 Apr;286:112555.
61. Trujillo M. Culture and the organization of psychiatric care. Psychiatr Clin North Am 2001 Sep;24(3):539–52.
62. Amowitz LL, Heisler M, Iacopino V. A population-based assessment of women's mental health and attitudes toward women's human rights in Afghanistan. J Womens Health (Larchmt). 2003;12(6):577–87.
63. Scholte WF, Olff M, Ventevogel P, et al. Mental health symptoms following war and repression in eastern Afghanistan. JAMA 2004;292(5):585–93.

64. Panter-Brick C, Eggerman M, Gonzalez V, et al. Violence, suffering, and mental health in Afghanistan: a school-based survey. Lancet 2009;374(9692):807–16.

65. Karam EG, Mneimneh ZN, Dimassi H, et al. Lifetime prevalence of mental disorders in Lebanon: first onset, treatment, and exposure to war. PLoS Med 2008; 5(4):e61.

66. Karliner LS, Jacobs EA, Chen AH, et al. Do professional interpreters improve clinical care for patients with limited English proficiency? A systematic review of the literature. Health Serv Res 2007;42(2):727–54.

67. Ramirez D, Engel KG, Tang TS. Language interpreter utilization in the emergency department setting: a clinical review. J Health Care Poor Underserved 2008; 19(2):352–62.

68. Riera A, Walker DM. The impact of race and ethnicity on care in the pediatric emergency department. Curr Opin Pediatr 2010;22(3):284–9.

69. Rojas CR, Coffin A, Taylor A, et al. Resident communication with patients and families preferring languages other than English. Hosp Pediatr 2023;13(6):480–91.

70. Maletsky KD, Worsley D, Tran Lopez K, et al. Communication experiences of caregivers using a language other than English on inpatient services. Hosp Pediatr 2023;13(6):471–9.

71. Rosenberg J, Chelemedos K, Luna L, et al. Gaps in clinical care and research inclusion for families speaking languages other than English. Hosp Pediatr 2023;13(6):e144–6.

72. Chen A, Demaestri S, Schweiberger K, et al. Inclusion of non-English-speaking participants in pediatric health research: a review. JAMA Pediatr 2023;177(1):81–8.

73. Collier VP. Age and rate of acquisition of second language for academic purposes. Tesol Q 1987;21(4):617–41.

74. Grunebaum MF, Mann JJ. Safe use of SSRIs in young adults: how strong is evidence for new suicide warning? Curr Psychiatr 2007;6(11):nihpa81089.

75. Johnson RAI. Refugee camp security: decreasing vulnerability through demographic controls. J Refug Stud 2011;24(1):23–46.

76. Lyles E, Hanquart B, Chlela L, et al. Health service access and utilization among syrian refugees and affected host communities in Lebanon. J Refug Stud 2018; 31(1):104–30.

77. McCauley E, Gudmundsen G, Schloredt K, et al. The adolescent behavioral activation program: adapting behavioral activation as a treatment for depression in adolescence. J Clin Child Adolesc Psychol 2016;45(3):291–304.

78. Wong MM, Brower KJ. The prospective relationship between sleep problems and suicidal behavior in the National Longitudinal Study of Adolescent Health. J Psychiatr Res 2012 Jul;46(7):953–9.

79. Gillespie S, Banegas J, Maxwell J, et al. Parenting interventions for refugees and forcibly displaced families: a systematic review. Clin Child Fam Psychol Rev 2022;25(2):395–412.

80. Zajac L, Raby KL, Dozier M. Receptive vocabulary development of children placed in foster care and children who remained with birth parents after involvement with child protective services. Child Maltreat 2019;24(1):107–12.

81. Luster T, Saltarelli AJ, Rana M, et al. The experiences of Sudanese unaccompanied minors in foster care. J Fam Psychol 2009;23(3):386–95.

82. Crea TM, Lopez A, Hasson RG, et al. Unaccompanied immigrant children in long term foster care: identifying needs and best practices from a child welfare perspective. Child Youth Serv Rev 2018;92:56–64.

83. Collier VP, Thomas WP. The astounding effectiveness of dual language education for all. NABE Journal of Research and Practice 2004;2(1):1–20.

84. Coates S, Gaensbauer TJ. Event trauma in early childhood: symptoms, assessment, intervention. Child Adolesc Psychiatr Clin N Am 2009;18(3):611–26 [published correction appears in Child Adolesc Psychiatr Clin N Am. 2009 Oct;18(4): 1027].
85. Bath H. The three pillars of trauma-informed care. Reclaiming Children and Youth 2008;17(3):17–21.
86. Lindsay S, King G, Klassen AF, et al. Working with immigrant families raising a child with a disability: challenges and recommendations for healthcare and community service providers. Disabil Rehabil 2012;34(23):2007–17.
87. Hill S, Petit J. The violent patient. Emerg Med Clin North Am 2000;18(2):301–15.
88. Gerson R, Malas N, Mroczkowski MM. Crisis in the emergency department: the evaluation and management of acute agitation in children and adolescents. Child Adolesc Psychiatr Clin N Am 2018;27(3):367–86.
89. McClure JM, Friedberg RD, Thordarson MA, et al. CBT express. Effective 15-minute techniques for treating children and adolescents. New York, NY: The Guildford Press; 2019.
90. Lieberman MD, Eisenberger NI, Crockett MJ, et al. Putting feelings into words. Psychol Sci 2007;18(5):421–8.
91. Hamari L, Konttila J, Merikukka M, et al. Parent support programmes for families who are immigrants: a scoping review. J Immigr Minor Health 2022;24(2):506–25.

Moving Forward in Mental Health Care for Refugee, Asylum-Seeking, and Undocumented Children

Social Determinants, Phased Approach to Care, and Advocacy

Keven Lee, PhD, MSc[a,b,*], Rachel Kronick, MD, MSc, FRCPC[a,b],
Diana Miconi, PhD, MA[c], Cécile Rousseau, MD, MSc[a]

KEYWORDS

- Refugee • Asylum seekers • Undocumented • Mental health • Phased approach
- Advocacy

KEY POINTS

- The mental health of refugee, asylum-seeking, or undocumented children, youth, and their families should be considered through a public health lens to redress the local and systemic inequities that directly and indirectly affect their well-being.
- A pyramidal approach to providing and implementing mental health services that acknowledge different and concurrent levels of needs should be prioritized to follow the child's developmental trajectories and changes in the resettlement process.
- An ecosocial perspective broadens our understanding of mental health distress by attending to the dynamic and circular interactions in-between the individual, family, community, historical, and sociopolitical dimensions.

INTRODUCTION

Since 1990, forced displacement has more than doubled, and, despite their resources, high-income countries welcome only a small proportion (24%) of those needing international protection, leaving low and middle-income countries (LMIC) to receive approximately three-quarters of those fleeing war or persecution.[1,2] An exception has been the response in Europe to the war in Ukraine, where Central Europe

[a] Division of Social and Transcultural Psychiatry, McGill University, 1033 Pine Avenue, Montreal, Quebec, Canada; [b] Lady Davis Institute, 3755 Côte Ste-Catherine Road, Montreal, Quebec; [c] Department of Educational Psychology and Adult Education, Université de Montréal, 90 Vincent D'Indy Avenue, Outremont, Montréal, QC, Canada
* Corresponding author.
E-mail address: Keven.lee@mcgill.ca

Child Adolesc Psychiatric Clin N Am 33 (2024) 237–250
https://doi.org/10.1016/j.chc.2023.09.007
1056-4993/24/© 2023 Elsevier Inc. All rights reserved.

received more than 8.2 million Ukrainian refugees, with Poland welcoming more than 1.6 million refugees alone. In the face of increasing climate disasters and protracted social unrest, forced displacement is expected to grow exponentially, raising new challenges for host societies to respond to the growing mental health and resettlement needs of migrants and refugees. In high-income countries, clinicians and policy-makers must urgently consider the social conditions and determinants that will promote these populations' well-being, recovery, and health, given current polarized discourses and racist and xenophobic sentiments jeopardizing migrants' sense of safety and integration.

This article focuses on how the present sociopolitical context influences the mental health concerns that forcibly displaced (ie, refugee, asylum-seeking, and undocumented) children face as they resettle in high-income host societies. First, we provide a brief overview of the determinants of mental health, highlighting the challenges emerging in the current political and socio-historical context. Second, we discuss principles guiding assessment and intervention to lessen the influence of the resettlement processes on mental health. Finally, we propose recommendations for structural change to promote health equity and human rights for sanctuary-seeking children, youth, and their families.

THE LANDSCAPE OF RISK AND PROTECTIVE FACTORS

Asylum seekers, refugees, and other precarious migrant families and children often arrive in a host society having already faced extreme forms of adversity only to meet new stressors and multiple forms of exclusion as they rebuild their lives. The risk and protective factors influencing mental health are usually organized temporally, distinguishing the determinants during premigration, migration, and postmigration.[3,4] Direct exposure to violence, loss, torture, and threat before migration are important determinants influencing the onset and persistence of mental health problems,[5] although research has increasingly pointed to the complex interaction between premigration trauma and postmigration adversity. Other perimigration factors that influence well-being include disruption of education, separation from family,[6] parental distress,[7] prolonged grief,[8] and harsh living conditions during the journey,[9] which is often marked by loss, insecurity, deprivation, and precarity.[10] In addition, such factors affect youth differently depending on their age and developmental stage. For adolescents, who are going through the developmental tasks of separation and individuation, migration and adaptation to a new environment can be particularly challenging.[11]

Although arrival in an ostensibly safe country might mark the beginning of stability and recovery for fleeing individuals, exposure to significant postmigratory stress may compound the effects of previous trauma.[12] Often, these stressors are constituted by forms of embodied exclusion resulting from structural inequities and restrictive immigration policies, manifesting as socioeconomic deprivation, including unemployment, substandard housing, as well as discrimination, racism, and social isolation.[4,13] Other challenges include language acquisition, cultural shock, and barriers to access education and services, particularly when host communities fail to facilitate equitable access.

Further, the precarity faced by children and families who do not have access to secure and permanent legal status, or who are undergoing protracted refugee claims process, is a known predictor of psychopathology.[14] In addition, policies of indefinite immigration detention, including those in the United States, Canada, Australia, and the United Kingdom, often result in parents' separation from children and are consistently found to be harmful to children.[15–18] The cumulative influence of previous trauma and its interaction with the postmigration stressors resulting from structural violence in a host society highlights the crucial role of newcomers' reception in host societies as a key determinant of mental health.[5,19]

An ecosocial perspective may be useful to clinicians because it elaborates on how cumulative and multilevel individual and structural factors facilitate or impede recovery, resettlement, and survival for children and families who have migrated. This ecosocial framing, developed by Bronfenbrenner, provides a viewfinder to capture a plurality of individual and collective experiences of families accounting for historical, social, political, and cultural factors that mediate and moderate the experiences of children and their communities. Although the previous paragraph refers to macrolevel determinants (eg, cultural, sociopolitical, and economic), an ecosocial approach also attends to the microlevel (ie, individual) and mesolevels that include factors such as family cohesion,[5] neighborhood climate, and the negotiation of one's cultural identity in a new context.[20] Although a sense of belonging to an ethnocultural group may be a protective factor by providing individual and collective resources and meaning,[21] it may have a dual effect because belonging to a marginalized ethnocultural group can lead to forms of systemic exclusion from host societies.[3,22]

Although not all migrant youth report mental health problems, the cumulative influences of previous trauma, migration, and structural violence can lead to the onset or aggravation of important, sometimes persistent,[11] psychological and psychiatric difficulties.[3] Earlier studies show higher rates of posttraumatic stress disorder (PTSD) among refugee and asylum-seeking youth.[23] Yet, there is a shift in focus from solely on PTSD to include a wider set of difficulties in the first 2 years following resettlement[24,25] such as stress-related disorders[26,27] and depression.[28,29] Further, meta-analyses show that the risk of psychotic disorders is potentially up to 5 times higher in both migrant adolescents and adults than in the general population[30,31] — with additional risks associated with forced migration.[32] These rates suggest that postmigration stressors such as discrimination, especially racism, play a role in the development of psychosis. Nonetheless, clinicians may also be attentive to the risks of misinterpreting responses to trauma and stress as psychotic.

The Healthy Migrant "Paradox"

Despite the multiple forms of adversity that children and youth face, studies have shown that they often adapt well to their new environments. Known as the "healthy immigrant effect" (HIE), this phenomenon reflects that migrant youth tend to have better health outcomes than their native-born peers.[33,34] This resilience is hypothesized to be linked with selection bias, the particular strengths of those migrating, better health habits, and parental expectations. The HIE also points to the human capacity for posttraumatic growth and transformation.[35] Interestingly, although refugees are considered to be an exception to the HIE, research has shown that some refugee children may fit this larger trend,[36] challenging representations of all refugees as vulnerable and burdensome. Current evidence points to the waning off of the HIE over time, although this has not been observed consistently across all host countries.[37] More longitudinal studies are needed to consider the short-term and long-term trajectories of mental health among refugee and asylum-seeking youth and how such trajectories can be shaped by the resettlement contexts.

Rise of Social Polarization: Being at Risk to Becoming a Risk

In the past decade, research on migrant children and youth often assumed that host societies provided refuge and safe resettlement for children who are seen as needing and deserving protection. Representations of migrants as vulnerable, particularly children, have progressively been replaced by their characterizations of children as potential threats to host societies. Indeed, the imaginary has shifted from migrant children *at risk* to migrant children *as risks*.[38] Children are portrayed as potentially dangerous and not as vulnerable and agentic,[4] resulting in migrant children and youth being considered, even by health-care workers, as "undeserving" of care[39] and potentially a threat to national security in parliamentary debates.[40] At the level of public opinion in Canada, for example, concerns regarding the legitimacy of refugees are increasing.[41] Antimigrant and refugee sentiments have not only resulted in more discrimination but also produced and legitimized restrictive migration policies, eroding migrants' rights to family unity, fair asylum hearings, protection from administrative detention, and limiting their access to health care and education.[42] Similar to majority groups, migrant and refugee communities may have a range of prejudices and internalized beliefs in terms of, but not limited to, gender, sexual orientation, caste, race, and religion. Intersectionality has been helpful in considering the cumulative effect of multiple forms of exclusion. It is not often, however, used to represent the wide heterogeneity within minority communities, which can, as any human group, be simultaneously victims and aggressors. In the present social polarization context, the emerging value clashes lead to complex situations that may be instrumentalized politically and require delicate ethical analysis.[43]

This evolving sociopolitical context and social polarization significantly influence the lives and health of migrant children and youth, straining social cohesion[44] and eroding migrants' sense of belonging.[45,46] The systemic subjugation of migrants was writ large in the United States under the Trump administration, leading to the separation of asylum-seeking children from their parents. Although less in the public eye, children continue to be detained in the United States and many asylum-seeking children live with the day-to-day fear of deportation.[47] Canada also restricted the benefits and protection granted to asylum-seekers by reducing access to health care under a previous government. While restoring health care, the current government has just expanded the Safe Third Country agreement to ensure fewer asylum-seekers can enter the country.

These othering processes have an institutional influence on the health and education systems, giving rise to important equity, diversity, and inclusion policies. Yet these initiatives have been criticized for their inability to address long-standing structural injustice, attitudinal changes, and for sparking backlash and sometimes exacerbating polarity. This polarization is reflected within school walls,[48] intensifying peer-to-peer tensions,[49,50] and teachers' discrimination toward newcomer youth.[51] Further, studies have shown how institutional policies and unconscious bias, often insidiously entangled, can erode the quality and accessibility of education and health care.[52,53] Rousseau and colleagues's[52] findings underscore that direct contact with refugees alone does not result in attitudinal changes of health-care providers. Transforming providers' views and treatment of migrants requires addressing representations of migration at the population level through institutional and governmental action as well as with policies that promote diversity, equity, and justice in health access and education.

CHALLENGES AND FUTURE DIRECTIONS IN ASSESSMENT AND INTERVENTION: TOWARD A PHASED APPROACH TO CARE

Despite the need for mental health services for migrant children, studies have shown that they are significantly underutilized or hard to access.[11,54] Current literature suggests that migrants are more inclined to use informal mental health support from either family members or friends and that the lack of access to interpreters, lack of cultural competence and humility of providers, stigmatization of mental illness, and the challenges of navigating health-care systems account for some barriers to mental health services for migrant youth and adults.[55]

Accessibility to mental health care should be considered at every stage of the resettlement process and requires the promotion of nonspecialized and community-based or school-based services as well as accessible specialized assessment and intervention. Addressing barriers faced by refugees, asylum-seekers, and undocumented families is also crucial, including access to subsidized, professional interpreters, support with transportation, and efforts to address stigma and navigation of complex health systems. Migrants without permanent status, such as asylum seekers and undocumented children, will also require special safeguards to ensure that their seeking health care is confidential, not putting them at risk for immigration enforcement. Ethical imperatives for clinicians always underline that physicians and care providers' chief responsibility is to the patient's best interests and protection from harm, and not to third-party actors, including immigration officials.[10,56]

Providing time-sensitive and culturally adapted care to migrant youth and their families becomes an even greater challenge in light of the present social tensions, anti-immigrant attitudes, and the lack of prioritization of migrant and refugee communities by some decision-makers. Although in North America, studies focus primarily on specialized treatments for psychiatric conditions, in LMIC, the focus is more on reestablishing a supportive environment to protect and promote the development of children and youth. Bridging these 2 literatures, the UK National Institute for Clinical Excellence (NICE) guidelines stress the importance of a phased approach to the treatment of stress-related disorders in refugee children.[11,57,58] Rousseau and Gagnon[24] propose 3 key moments in young people's resettlement processes (arrival, first 2 years, and long-term) to guide professionals in the assessment and provision of intervention that accounts for the evolving needs and challenges faced by this population over time.

Phase One: Arrival

On arrival, children and youth may present more acute stress-related symptoms linked to premigration and perimigration experiences and perceived insecurity in the host country combined with their specific developmental needs and the demands of the initial adjustment process. Yet, because of positive expectations conveyed by the parents and community toward the host country, some children and youth might present with initial relief of symptoms on arrival, although this does not foreclose the potential for a later deterioration of their mental health. Hence, it remains important for clinicians to monitor child and family well-being longitudinally. At this stage, interventions should focus on addressing basic needs and on restoring some sense of safety and normalcy, including access to school and housing and supporting asylum seekers in their refugee claim.[11] While working with this population, clinicians should be alert to issues of trust and distrust and seek to accurately reassure asylum seekers and refugees of their confidentiality and that receiving care will not jeopardize their status. Clinicians should advocate for the youth and their families so that their basic needs are met, and in cases where legislation or policy threatens confidential health care or access to services, ethical guidelines suggest that patients' best interests always be prioritized over other interests.[59] Nonspecific interventions should also focus on the establishment of meaningful connections within families and communities, given heightened family stress during this period and the social isolation and exclusion often experienced.

Psychological first-aid[60,61] (PFA) is a promising approach that can be delivered by clinicians and nonclinicians alike, which aims to lessen the emotional distress experienced by those affected by crises to prevent short-term and long-term mental health consequences through supportive and context-adapted intervention. PFA is structured around 5 core tenets (*safety, calming, connectedness, self-efficacy,* and *hope*) to foster the restoration of normalcy while also screening for further needs. Community and schools are well-suited environments for PFA and have been used with migrant youth to foster emotional safety.[11,62–65] Schools in particular are in a privileged position to offer such universal and supportive interventions because they are the primary setting of the acculturation process, becoming a natural bridge between migrant families and the host culture without the stigma of mental health services.[24,66,67] There is growing evidence supporting the positive influence of school-based interventions on mental health outcomes for migrant youth[65,68] through providing positive collective experiences to foster belonging[69] and group cohesion.[70] Although schools are often considered ideal naturalistic settings to reestablish safety and normalcy, there is a need for more ecological approaches that go beyond school and classroom environments to build bridges with local communities.[24,50,71,72]

Although the NICE guidelines suggest "the routine use of a validated, brief screening instrument for PTSD as part of any comprehensive physical and mental health screen"[58] of refugees and asylum seekers, there is no evidence of added benefit of systematic screening.[11] Canadian guidelines on Immigrant and Refugee Health[57] emphasize that early screening for PTSD should be avoided as potentially harmful. Formal early mental health assessments may be perceived as intrusive and stigmatizing and be put on hold, when possible, until after initial stabilization and establishing trusting relationships. Building trusting relationships takes time and demands both an ongoing exercise of cultural humility from the clinician and the establishment of strong partnerships with community organizations, leaders, and interpreters who may play the crucial role of cultural brokers and mediators. Nonspecific interventions such as PFA concurrently offer the opportunity to provide timely support for migrant youth's mental health and to assess for further needs while avoiding the risks of stigma and intrusion associated with clinical assessments.[60] Zealous and well-intentioned efforts to perform cognitive testing on migrant children soon after arrival, for example, can result in invalid results with highly negative consequences for children, such as placement in special education. Very often, acute stress symptoms disappear without individualized treatment once a sense of safety is established.[11] Nonetheless, clinicians should be attentive to any behavioral, emotional, cognitive, or unexplained medical symptoms, which may be related to exposure to traumatic events or the toxic stress of resettlement.

Phase Two: the First 2 Years Postresettlement in Host Societies

In approximately the first 2 years of resettlement, children who continue to display a high level of distress or significant impairment will require access to clinical assessment and more specialized educational and mental health services. Although some youth may need clinical and specialized care before, after 2 years, most children or youth will have had enough time to learn the language and adapt, to some degree, to their new environment thus moving beyond the normal and initial upheaval associated with a stressful adaptation process. For some children, this initial period of adaptation will be shorter or longer. In all cases, the assessment should follow an ecosocial approach to better understand distress, symptoms, and families' lifeworlds.[3,73,74] The ecosocial approach conceptualizes mental health as the dynamic and circular interactions of individuals, family, and community factors intersecting with larger structures and systems.[75–77] This perspective broadens our conceptualizations of mental disorders as more than individual psychopathology to acknowledge how social, cultural, and political contexts continue to shape experiences and suffering.[3]

Clinicians can begin to address unresolved grief, trauma, and resettlement difficulties, including family issues such as parental depression, conflicts in the family, and social exclusion. Importantly, clinicians must be aware that some migrant families will remain in situations of extreme precarity longer than 2 years after arrival either because they are undocumented, have not had their asylum claims adjudicated, or are facing protracted separations from family members who may still face ongoing threats to their safety. For these families, clinicians may address their suffering through solidarity and advocacy for their safety, including writing evaluation reports to support their asylum claim or reunion with family members seeking protection.[78,79] The first 2 years are also crucial in assessing developmental, learning, and speech delays, which may be difficult to detect earlier when there is not yet mastery of the host country's language. Special attention should be given to toddlers whose needs often remain undetected because their verbal expression is limited and because they communicate their distress through nonspecific symptoms. This may be combined with the potential for overburdened parents minimizing their children's distress.

During the clinical encounter, historical and social determinants that shape suffering and meaning will also influence the families' relationship with clinicians. Exposure to organized, interpersonal, and structural violence has insidious and long-lasting effects that may challenge the therapeutic alliance. For many, silence and distrust are highly normative and adaptive responses to past adversity. Clinicians must carefully attend to power dynamics inherent in clinical encounters that cannot be *solved* or erased and navigate the therapeutic process in ways that allow the building of trust and eventual modulated disclosure—without being directive and assuming that avoidance and distrust are purely pathologic. It is suggested that clinicians should hone an approach of *cultural humility*,[80] following the youth and families' own pace and survival strategies that will foster trust. The Cultural Formulation Interview (CFI), presented below, can be a useful tool for clinicians to cultivate cultural humility. Rousseau and colleagues[81] suggest a "safe enough" approach to cultural safety, acknowledging the limits of health-care workers' ability to ensure safety and how distress and discomfort are part of the clinical process. It further stresses that historical oppression cannot be swiftly erased and necessitates concerted and continuous efforts.

Ultimately, the assessment process should be viewed as an unfolding process of witnessing, accompaniment, and building solidarity with a family to help facilitate their pathway to safety, survival, and recovery.[3,24] The Adaption and Development after Persecution and Trauma (ADAPT) model developed by Silove,[82] initially designed for individuals and communities who have undergone mass conflict, is a useful ecosocial framework to support the assessment and treatment process. ADAPT identifies 5 core psychosocial pillars (*safety and security*; *interpersonal bonds and networks*; *justice*; *roles and identities*; *and existential meaning and coherence*) that must be reestablished for individuals and collectives to regain "mental equilibrium"[83] after the shattering of their psychosocial worlds. Kronick and colleagues propose an applied approach to the ADAPT model that can help guide assessment and intervention when working with migrants.[3]

Phase Three: Long-Term Adaptation

In the third and long-term phase, in which youth and families are resettled, clinicians must keep nurturing their cultural humility and be alert to cultural, historical, and contextual factors that remain challenging and might trigger the persistence or reactivation of previous trauma. In some cases, the resettlement context is chronically unsafe with insecure status being a particularly salient risk.[14] At times, cumulative toxic stress warrants a diagnosis of complex PTSD (C-PTSD), which includes, in addition to the classic PTSD symptoms, the triad of emotional dysregulation, changes in self-concept, and disturbances in relational functioning,[84] and that underlines the exposure to a prolonged period of helplessness, the loss of important supporting relationships in combination with traumatic events. Although C-PTSD is included in the stress-based disorders of the International Classification of Diseases 11th Revision (ICD-11), it does not yet have recognition in the Diagnostic and statistical manual of mental disorders (DSM-5-TR). Researchers have noted that C-PTSD is sometimes misdiagnosed as borderline personality disorder or as conduct disorder preventing youth from getting the specific treatment they need.[85]

The CFI included in the DSM-5-TR[86] is a useful assessment tool for clinicians that can help with differential diagnosis and case formulation. Its core module can help guide the exploration of the cultural dimensions that can be related to mental health disorders, such as patients' idioms of distress, explanatory models, cultural factors related to their psychosocial environment, and the relationship with the clinician. In addition, the CFI has supplemental modules to be used with migrant populations, children, and adolescents.

Although a review of available and effective interventions with migrant children and youth goes beyond the scope of the current article (see Kronick[10] and colleagues[3] for overviews), it is important that clinicians consider the youth's preferences and pace in the choice of interventions.[24] Further, within an ecosocial approach, clinicians should acknowledge and, whenever possible, address systemic injustices, discrimination, and violence that migrant children and youth may experience. This involves advocacy at the individual patient level, such as supporting access to safe housing, financial resources, and asylum, as well as at the structural level, which includes intersectoral advocacy for changes in policies regarding care delivery, prohibiting practices of immigration detention, and advancing clinical training.[87,88]

CLINICAL WORK AND ADVOCACY

Alongside a phased approach, host societies must view the mental health of migrant youth through structural and public health lenses.[3,11,70] Efforts to redress systemic inequity and the structural determinants of mental health are essential given current sociopolitical realities and climate. Considering the various and concurrent needs of migrant youth, a pyramidal model of providing mental health care that acknowledges different levels of services and their integrated implementation should be prioritized. A pyramidal model also emphasizes the critical role of approaching mental health from a public health perspective in providing basic needs and safety at its foundation[3]— whether it relates to providing access to legal counsel, fair asylum proceedings, secure housing, or access to a myriad of services, including subsidized daycare, which can pave a pathway to family security.

The Interagency Standing Committee,[89] of the United Nations, proposes a model in which our first duty is to advocate for and foster a social context that provides basic needs and protects children and their families from the harms of structural violence, leaving specialized clinical services (ie, mental health care by mental health specialists) as a *last resort*. The next level of interventions and services should aim at strengthening existing relationships at the family and community levels as well as fostering new bonds to mitigate the harmful effects of social isolation on mental health and well-being. Interventions should be nonspecialized and offered in the community.[70] The penultimate tier should focus on individual interventions provided by community workers and mental health professionals in primary care or trusted community settings. Finally, the top tier consists of specialized psychological or psychiatric interventions.

It is imperative that services are delivered concurrently and flexibly, following youth's developmental trajectories and changes in the resettlement process, a process in which uncertainty is often ubiquitous. This approach stresses the importance of bringing together multisector partners, including clinicians, community workers, scholars, and decision-makers, to support migrant youth and advocate for care that transcends a focus on individuals' symptoms to encompass health promotion and prevention, thus redressing inherent social and health inequalities.[11,36,90] As much as possible, clinicians should connect and collaborate with local communities and community organizations to support and accompany their patients and better respond do their needs. Centering the voices of migrant children and families is also crucial for the development of future research, interventions, and policies. Clinical-level and structural advocacy position us in roles of accompaniment in which we may act in solidarity *with* forcibly displaced migrants to address social suffering and the social determinants that shape families' trajectories.

CLINICS CARE POINTS

- Assessment and intervention for refugee, asylum-seeking, and undocumented children, youth, and families should follow a phased-approach to care.

- An ecosocial approach can help articulate and better respond to social suffering and distress, integrating individual-level determinants with the social, cultural, and political context.

- In the first 2 years of resettlement, nonspecific interventions to restore safety and foster the development of meaningful connections should be prioritized.

- School-based and community-based interventions following a PFA approach are promising to foster the well-being of refugee, asylum-seeking, and undocumented children, youth, and families.

- Specialized psychological and psychiatric interventions should be seen as a last resort, whereas policy and intervention to address structural violence and inequity are primary.

- Clinicians should advocate for children's and families' best interests and protection at all resettlement phases.

DISCLOSURE

The authors want to acknowledge the Canadian Institute for Health Research (grant number: 468562).

REFERENCES

1. UNHRC. Refugee Data Finder. Accessed Dec. 2022, https://www.unhcr.org/refugee-statistics/
2. McAuliffe M, Triandafyllidou A, editors. World migration report 2022. Geneva: International Organization for Migration (IOM); 2021. p. 522.
3. Kronick R, Jarvis GE, Kirmayer LJ. Migration mental health: immigrants, refugees and displaced persons. In: Tasman A, Riba MB, Schutze T, editors. Tasman textbook of psychiatry. 5th edition. Cham: Springer; 2023. p. 1–31. *In press*.

4. Hynie M. The social determinants of refugee mental health in the post-migration context: a critical review. Can J Psychiatr 2018;63(5):297–303.

5. Fazel M, Reed RV, Panter-Brick C, et al. Mental health of displaced and refugee children resettled in high-income countries: risk and protective factors. Lancet 2012;379(9812):266–82.

6. De Haene L, Rousseau C, editors. Working with refugee families: trauma and exile in family relationships. Cambridge, United Kingdom: Cambridge University Press; 2020. p. 340.

7. Eruyar S, Maltby J, Vostanis P. Mental health problems of Syrian refugee children: the role of parental factors. Eur Child Adolesc Psychiatry 2018;27(4):401–9.

8. Bryant RA, Edwards B, Creamer M, et al. Prolonged grief in refugees, parenting behaviour and children's mental health. Aust N Z J Psychiatr 2021;55(9):863–73.

9. Van de Wiel W, Castillo-Laborde C, Francisco Urzúa I, et al. Mental health consequences of long-term stays in refugee camps: preliminary evidence from Moria. BMC Publ Health 2021;21(1):1–10.

10. Kronick R. Mental health of refugees and asylum seekers: assessment and intervention. Can J Psychiatr 2018;63(5):290–6.

11. Rousseau C, Frounfelker RL. Mental health needs and services for migrants: an overview for primary care providers. J Trav Med 2019;26(2).

12. Jannesari S, Hatch S, Prina M, et al. Post-migration social–environmental factors associated with mental health problems among asylum seekers: a systematic review. J Immigr Minority Health 2020;22:1055–64.

13. Gleeson C, Frost R, Sherwood L, et al. Post-migration factors and mental health outcomes in asylum-seeking and refugee populations: a systematic review. Eur J Psychotraumatol 2020;11(1):1793567.

14. Ratnamohan L, Silove D, Mares S, et al. Breaching the family walls: modelling the impact of prolonged visa insecurity on asylum-seeking children. Aust N Z J Psychiatr 2023;1–10.

15. Kronick R, Rousseau C, Cleveland J. Asylum-seeking children's experiences of detention in Canada: a qualitative study. Am J Orthopsychiatry 2015;85(3):287–94.

16. MacLean SA, Agyeman PO, Walther J, et al. Mental health of children held at a United States immigration detention center. Soc Sci Med 2019;230:303–8.

17. von Werthern M, Robjant K, Chui Z, et al. The impact of immigration detention on mental health: a systematic review. BMC Psychiatr 2018;18(1):1–19.

18. Mares S. Mental health consequences of detaining children and families who seek asylum: a scoping review. Eur Child Adolesc Psychiatr 2021;30(10):1615–39.

19. Measham T, Heidenreich-Dutray F, Rousseau C, et al. Cultural consultation in child psychiatry. In: Kirmayer LJ, Guzder J, Rousseau C, editors. Cultural consultation: encountering the other in mental health care. New York: Springer; 2014. p. 71–87.

20. Choy B, Arunachalam K, Gupta S, et al. Systematic review: acculturation strategies and their impact on the mental health of migrant populations. Public Health in Practice 2021;2:100069.

21. Bécares L, Dewey ME, Das-Munshi J. Ethnic density effects for adult mental health: systematic review and meta-analysis of international studies. Psychol Med 2018;48(12):2054–72.

22. Jurcik T, Sunohara M, Yakobov E, et al. Acculturation and adjustment of migrants reporting trauma: the contextual effects of perceived ethnic density. J Community Psychol 2019;47(6):1313–28.

23. El Baba R, Colucci E. Post-traumatic stress disorders, depression, and anxiety in unaccompanied refugee minors exposed to war-related trauma: a systematic review. International Journal of Culture and Mental Health 2018;11(2):194–207.

24. Rousseau C, Gagnon MM. Intervening to address the impact of stress and trauma on refugee children and adolescents resettled in high-income countries. In: Song SJ, Ventevogel P, editors. Child, adolescent and Family refugee mental health: a global perspective. Cham: Springer International Publishing; 2020. p. 151–63.

25. Blackmore R, Gray KM, Boyle JA, et al. Systematic review and meta-analysis: the prevalence of mental illness in child and adolescent refugees and asylum seekers. J Am Acad Child Adolesc Psychiatr 2020;59(6):705–14.

26. Betancourt TS, Newnham EA, Birman D, et al. Comparing trauma exposure, mental health needs, and service utilization across clinical samples of refugee, immigrant, and US-origin children. J Trauma Stress 2017;30(3):209–18.

27. Hassan G, Ventevogel P, Jefee-Bahloul H, et al. Mental health and psychosocial wellbeing of Syrians affected by armed conflict. Epidemiol Psychiatr Sci 2016; 25(2):129–41.

28. Gagné MÈ, Marcotte D, Fortin LL. 'impact de la dépression et de l'expérience scolaire sur le décrochage scolaire des adolescents. Canadian Journal of Education/Revue canadienne de l'éducation 2011;34(2):77–92.

29. Bogic M, Njoku A, Priebe S. Long-term mental health of war-refugees: a systematic literature review. BMC Int Health Hum Right 2015;15:1.

30. Jongsma HE, Karlsen S, Kirkbride JB, et al. Understanding the excess psychosis risk in ethnic minorities: the impact of structure and identity. Soc Psychiatr Psychiatr Epidemiol 2021;56(11):1913–21.

31. Selten JP, Van Der Ven E, Termorshuizen F. Migration and psychosis: a meta-analysis of incidence studies. Psychol Med 2020;50(2):303–13.

32. Brandt L, Henssler J, Müller M, et al. Risk of psychosis among refugees: a systematic review and meta-analysis. JAMA Psychiatr 2019;76(11):1133–40.

33. Vang ZM, Sigouin J, Flenon A, et al. Are immigrants healthier than native-born Canadians? A systematic review of the healthy immigrant effect in Canada. Ethn Health 2017;22(3):209–41.

34. Constant AF, García-Muñoz T, Neuman S, et al. A "healthy immigrant effect" or a "sick immigrant effect"? Selection and policies matter. Eur J Health Econ 2018;19: 103–21.

35. Cohen K, Collens P. The impact of trauma work on trauma workers: a metasynthesis on vicarious trauma and vicarious posttraumatic growth. Psychological Trauma: Theory, Research, Practice, and Policy 2013;5(6):570.

36. Rousseau C. Addressing mental health needs of refuges. Canadian journal of psychiatry. Rev Canad Psychiatr 2018;63(5):287–9.

37. Elshahat S, Moffat T, Newbold KB. Understanding the healthy immigrant effect in the context of mental health challenges: a systematic critical review. J Immigr Minority Health 2022;24(6):1564–79.

38. Rousseau C. Continuity and shifts in contemporary refugee history. In: Wenzel T, Drożdek B, editors. An uncertain safety: integrative health care for the 21st century refugees. Cham: Springer; 2019. v-ix.

39. Vanthuyne K, Meloni F, Ruiz-Casares M, et al. Health workers' perceptions of access to care for children and pregnant women with precarious immigration status: health as a right or a privilege? Soc Sci Med 2013;93:78–85.

40. Kronick R, Rousseau C. Rights, compassion and invisible children: a critical discourse analysis of the parliamentary debates on the mandatory detention of migrant children in Canada. J Refug Stud 2015;28(4):544–69.

41. The Environics Institute for Survey Research, Century Initiative. Canadian public opinion about immigration and refugees - Fall 2022. 2022.

42. Samari G, Alcalá HE, Sharif MZ. Islamophobia, health, and public health: a systematic literature review. American Journal of Public Health 2018;108(6):e1–9.

43. Rousseau C, Machouf A. A preventive pilot project addressing multiethnic tensions in the wake of the Iraq war. Am J Orthopsychiatry 2005;75(4):466–74.

44. Hickman MJ, Mai N. Migration and social cohesion: appraising the resilience of place in London. Popul Space Place 2015;21(5):421–32.

45. Rousseau C, Measham T, Nadeau L. Addressing trauma in collaborative mental health care for refugee children. Clin Child Psychol Psychiatr 2013;18(1):121–36.

46. Siriwardhana C, Ali SS, Roberts B, et al. A systematic review of resilience and mental health outcomes of conflict-driven adult forced migrants. Conflict Health 2014;8(1):1–14.

47. Cervantes W, Ullrich R, Matthews H. Our Children's Fear: Immigration Policy's Effects on Young Children. Washington. 2018.

48. Rousseau C, Beauregard C, Michalon-Brodeur V. Penser la prévention pour les enfants réfugiés et immigrants: quand altérité et souffrance sociale se conjuguent. In: Dorais M, editor. Prévenir. Quebec: Presse de l'Université Laval; 2017.

49. Papazian-Zohrabian G, Mamprin C, Lemire V, et al. Le milieu scolaire québécois face aux défis de l'accueil des élèves réfugiés : quels enjeux pour la gouvernance scolaire et la formation des intervenants scolaires? Educ Francoph 2018;46(2):208–29.

50. Archambault I, Audet G, Borri-Anadon C, Hirsch S, Tardif-Grenier K. L'impact du climat interculturel des établissements sur la réussite éducative des élèves issus de l'immigration. Washington. 2019.

51. Becker B, Raschke E, Vieluf S, et al. Teaching refugee students: the role of teachers' attitudes towards cultural diversity. Teachers and Teaching 2023;29(4): 369–83.

52. Rousseau C, Oulhote Y, Ruiz-Casares M, et al. Encouraging understanding or increasing prejudices: a cross-sectional survey of institutional influence on health personnel attitudes about refugee claimants' access to health care. PLoS One 2017;12(2):e0170910.

53. Ruiz-Casares M, Rousseau C, Laurin-Lamothe A, et al. Access to health care for undocumented migrant children and pregnant women: the paradox between values and attitudes of health care professionals. Matern Child Health J 2013; 17:292–8.

54. Sarría-Santamera A, Hijas-Gómez AI, Carmona R, et al. A systematic review of the use of health services by immigrants and native populations. Publ Health Rev 2016;37(1):1–29.

55. Mohammadifirouzeh M, Oh KM, Basnyat I, et al. Factors associated with professional mental help-seeking among us immigrants: a systematic review. J Immigr Minority Health 2023;1–19.

56. Physicians for Human Rights. Dual loyalties: the challenges of providing professional health care to immigration detainees. 2011;

57. Rousseau C, Pottie K, Thombs BD, et al. Post traumatic stress disorder: evidence review for newly arriving immigrants and refugees. Guidelines for immigrant health, Canadian Collaboration for Immigrant and Refugee Health, Appendix 11. Can Med Assoc 2011.

58. National Institute for Health and Care Excellence. Post-traumatic stress disorder. London: NICE guideline; 2018.
59. Physicians for Human Rights. Dual Loyalty & Human Rights In Health Professional Practice: Proposed Guidelines & Institutional Mechanisms. 2003.
60. World Health Organization. Psychological first aid: guide for field workers. Geneva: World Health Organization; 2011.
61. Feldman R, Vengrober A. Posttraumatic stress disorder in infants and young children exposed to war-related trauma. J Am Acad Child Adolesc Psychiatr 2011; 50(7):645–58.
62. de Freitas Girardi J, Miconi D, Lyke C, et al. Creative expression workshops as psychological first aid (Pfa) for asylum-seeking children: an exploratory study in temporary shelters in Montreal. Clin Child Psychol Psychiatr 2020;25(2): 483–93.
63. Rousseau C, Miconi D. Welcoming refugee children: the role of psychological first aid interventions. Psynopsis 2018;40(4):8–9.
64. Beauregard C, Rousseau C, Benoit M, et al. Creating a safe space during classroom-based sandplay workshops for immigrant and refugee preschool children. J Creativ Ment Health 2022;1–17. https://doi.org/10.1080/15401383.2022. 2076001.
65. Fazel M, Betancourt TS. Preventive mental health interventions for refugee children and adolescents in high-income settings. Lancet Child & Adolescent Health 2018;2(2):121–32.
66. Birman D, Weinstein T, Chan W, et al. Immigrant youth in US schools: opportunities for prevention. Prev Res 2007;14(4):14–7.
67. Beehler S, Birman D, Campbell R. The effectiveness of cultural adjustment and trauma services (CATS): generating practice-based evidence on a comprehensive, school-based mental health intervention for immigrant youth. Am J Community Psychol 2012;50:155–68.
68. Brown RC, Witt A, Fegert JM, et al. Psychosocial interventions for children and adolescents after man-made and natural disasters: a meta-analysis and systematic review. Psychol Med 2017;47(11):1893–905.
69. Kia-Keating M, Ellis BH. Belonging and connection to school in resettlement: young refugees, school belonging, and psychosocial adjustment. Clin Child Psychol Psychiatr 2007;12(1):29–43.
70. Miconi D, Rousseau C. Children and vulnerable groups services. In: Bhugra D, editor. Oxford textbook of migrant psychiatry. New York: Oxford University Press; 2021. p. 413–22.
71. Fazel M, Hoagwood K. School mental health: integrating young people's voices to shift the paradigm. Lancet Child and Adolescent Health 2021;5(3):156–7.
72. Podar MD, Frețian AM, Demir Z, et al. How schools in Germany shape and impact the lives of adolescent refugees in terms of mental health and social mobility. SSM-Population Health 2022;19:101169.
73. Miller KE, Rasmussen A. The mental health of civilians displaced by armed conflict: an ecological model of refugee distress. Epidemiol Psychiatr Sci 2017;26(2): 129–38.
74. Scharpf F, Kaltenbach E, Nickerson A, et al. A systematic review of socio-ecological factors contributing to risk and protection of the mental health of refugee children and adolescents. Clin Psychol Rev 2021;83:101930.
75. Kirmayer LJ, Gómez-Carrillo A. Culturally responsive clinical psychology and psychiatry: an ecosocial approach. In: Maerrcher A, Haim E, Kirmayer LJ, editors. Cultural clinical psychology and PTSD. Boston, MA: Hogrefe; 2019. p. 3–21.

76. Gómez-Carrillo A, Kirmayer LJ. A cultural-ecosocial systems view for psychiatry. Front Psychiatr 2023;14:486.
77. Krieger N. Ecosocial theory, embodied truths, and the people's health. New York, NY: Oxford University Press; 2021.
78. Haas BM. "Asylum is the most powerful medicine": navigating therapeutic interventions in limbo. Cult Med Psychiatr 2021;45(2):193–217.
79. Stein D, Raju P, Andermann L. Diagnosis as advocacy: medico-legal reports in refugee family care. In: De Haene L, Rousseau C, editors. Working with refugee families: trauma and exile in family relationships. Cambridge, United Kingdom: Cambridge University Press; 2020. p. 232–48.
80. Trinh N-H, Jahan AB, Chen JA. Moving from cultural competence to cultural humility in psychiatric education. Psychiatr Clin 2021;44(2):149–57.
81. Rousseau C, Gomez-Carrillo A, Cénat JM. Safe enough? Rethinking the concept of cultural safety in healthcare and training. Br J Psychiatry: J Ment Sci 2022; 221(4):587–8.
82. Silove D. Adaptation, ecosocial safety signals, and the trajectory of PTSD. In: Kirmayer LJ, Lemelson R, Barad M, editors. Understanding trauma: integrating biological, psychological and cultural perspectives. Cambridge, United Kingdom: Cambridge University Press; 2007. p. 242–58.
83. Silove D, Ventevogel P, Rees S. The contemporary refugee crisis: an overview of mental health challenges. World Psychiatr 2017;16(2):130–9.
84. Brewin CR, Cloitre M, Hyland P, et al. A review of current evidence regarding the ICD-11 proposals for diagnosing PTSD and complex PTSD. Clin Psychol Rev 2017;58:1–15.
85. Cloitre M, Garvert DW, Weiss B, et al. Distinguishing PTSD, complex PTSD, and borderline personality disorder: a latent class analysis. Eur J Psychotraumatol 2014;5(1):25097.
86. Lewis-Fernández R, Aggarwal NK, Hinton L, et al, editors. The DSM-5 handbook on the cultural formulation interview. Washington: American Psychiatric Publishing; 2016. p. 330.
87. Kirmayer LJ, Kronick R, Rousseau C. Advocacy as key to structural competency in psychiatry. JAMA Psychiatr 2018;75(2):119–20.
88. Jarvis GE, Andermann L, Ayonrinde OA, et al. Taking action on racism and structural violence in psychiatric training and clinical practice. Can J Psychiatr 2023; 0(0). https://doi.org/10.1177/07067437231166985.
89. IASC Reference Group for Mental Health and Psychosocial Support in Emergency Settings. Mental Health and Psychosocial Support in Humanitarian Emergencies: What Should Humanitarian Health Actor Know? 2010.
90. Cleveland J, Rousseau C, Guzder J. Cultural consultation for refugees. In: Kirmayer LJ, Guzder J, Rousseau C, editors. Cultural consultation: encountering the other in mental health care. New York: Springer; 2013. p. 245–68.

Acculturating Systems of Care to Ensure Healthy Futures for Latine Migrant Youth

Leeallie Pearl Carter, MD

KEYWORDS

- Migrant • Youth • Systems of care • Acculturation

KEY POINTS

- Just as migrant youth go through a process of acculturating to a new culture on arrival in the United States, systems of care may also adapt in a variety of ways.
- Integrative strategies of acculturation place value on prioritizing connection to both cultures, have evidence for supporting mental health outcomes in immigrants, and may prove a model for systems to follow in their adaptive process.
- Examples of integrative adaptations of systems of care may include challenging misinformation, celebrating heritage days, including cultural references in education, hiring bicultural and bilingual staff, and pursuing policy changes to expand accessibility to services.

INTRODUCTION

Migration is a natural, constantly evolving phenomenon impacting all parts of the globe, across species.[1] In the western hemisphere, trade has long connected what we currently call North, Central, South America, and the Caribbean via land, river, and coastal migratory routes.[2] Although movement of individuals from across the Americas into what is currently known as the United States is not new, the number of immigrants has steadily risen since the 1970s, with complex political and economic drivers.[3] Since the 1970s, immigration trends in the United States have also begun a return to a greater percentage of immigrants coming from the Americas as opposed to Europe, with increases in African and Asian immigration as well.[3] In fact, US census data estimate one in six Americans are currently coded as Hispanic and this is anticipated to increase to one in three by the year 2060, with Hispanic defined as "a person of Cuban, Mexican, Puerto Rican, South or Central American or other Spanish culture."[4] Hispanic youth made up 26% of children in the United States in 2020 census data with a sizable minority arriving during childhood.[5]

Mountain Area Health Education Center in Asheville, NC in partnership with the University of North Carolina-Chapel Hill, 125 Hendersonville Road, Asheville, NC 28803, USA
E-mail address: leealliecarter@gmail.com

Child Adolesc Psychiatric Clin N Am 33 (2024) 251–261
https://doi.org/10.1016/j.chc.2023.10.004
childpsych.theclinics.com
1056-4993/24/© 2023 Elsevier Inc. All rights reserved.

When children and families arrive and at times even before arrival, they begin engaging in various systems of care within the United States. Systems of care refer to the community programs and networks that provide services to children and families such as education, mental health care, primary health care, child welfare, immigration, developmental disabilities, substance use treatment, and juvenile justice systems.[6] Collaboration across systems strengthens the work that any individual partner is providing, which is why the American Academy of Child and Adolescent Psychiatrists, the American Academy of Pediatrics, the US Department of Health and Human Services, and others are increasingly offering training and resources to improve our collective ability to partner in ways that increase access to coordinated high-quality and culturally appropriate services.[7-9]

In this article, the author explores the experience of one young Guatemalan boy from the perspective of a resident engaging across systems to ensure a coordinated response to his mental health needs. The current roles of various systems of care in the lives of migrant youth will be highlighted, with a primary focus on health care and education systems. The typical focus on encouraging change within migrant populations will be challenged and opportunities for the systems themselves to rapidly shift will be asserted. This aims to ensure healthy environments and access to culturally appropriate early intervention for Latine migrant youth experiencing mental and emotional distress. The author reviews the experiences of pre and postmigration that increase the risk for mental disorders in migrant youth generally and may impact their relationship to engagement with systems of care. A note on terms—Hispanic and Latine, a gender-neutral term broadly encompassing people of Latin American descent, will be used interchangeably. Interpersonally, we use the term (Latin/o/a/x/e, Hispanic, country of origin, indigenous nation, and so forth) preferred by the individual and encourage others to do the same.

Questions to consider are included to invite reflection on personal and systems impacts to acculturative stress.

LATINE MIGRANT YOUTH: AN ABBREVIATED HISTORY

Consider the patient who inspired the exploration contained within this article: "Luis" is a 14-year-old K'iche' Guatemalan boy who immigrated to the United States at age 10 and had no significant past medical or psychiatric history when he presented to the emergency department voluntarily with his father at the urgence of a school nurse following several months of inability to establish outpatient primary or psychiatric care in the setting of increasing social withdrawal, decreased intake, mutism, and most recently, urinary incontinence and nose bleeding. He was admitted for severe major depressive disorder with malignant catatonia and ultimately required a greater than 100 day stay for enteral nutrition, electroconvulsive therapy (ECT), and medication initiation.

A reflection from a psychiatric resident in North Carolina on caring for Luis:

I had met a particular patient in the hospital, coincidentally, on their last day of a very long hospitalization. This is a child who spent months decompensating physically due to low mood. Both the family and school found him over time to be falling behind academically with increasingly isolative behaviors. Eventually, the child became severely malnourished to the point of medical emergency. This child spent months in a hospital with no clear understanding of what triggered a depression that developed into catatonia. There was a lot of speculation regarding family ability to care for their child, psychosis and possible abuse. With only speculation, this child decompensated after discharge, to the point where re-hospitalization was necessary. It wasn't until I was able to develop a consistent outpatient relationship with this child that it became clear acculturation was the biggest contributor to their mood. Without collaborative care involving the education, primary healthcare, mental healthcare, immigration, child welfare, and disabilities systems, progress would not be made. Almost weekly meetings were conducted across systems to coordinate care for this child's complex needs. During these sessions, it became clear that signs of this child struggling with their transition to America were missed early on. The question that follows me is whether the severity of his illness may have been prevented had our systems of care more seamlessly provided coordinated, culturally appropriate services from symptom onset.

—Sonia Koul, PGY-2

PREMIGRATION FACTORS

Before considering opportunities to better support children like Luis within our current systems of care, let us briefly consider the historical factors contributing to complex mental health consequences for Latine youth today. European and Anglo-American powers have engaged in centuries of colonization throughout Latin America.[10] International involvement continues up to current times and we can use Nicaragua to illustrate this, as the National Hispanic and Latino Mental Health Technology Transfer Center Network describes in their work on adapting evidence-based practices for Latine youth:

For example, consider that from 1981 to 1990, in a fight against communism, the US intervened in Nicaragua to combat the influence of communism, a rising Marxist governmental regime. This intervention included the economic funding and tactical training of rebel militant groups (Contras) in Nicaragua that committed mass terrorist attacks and human rights violations against Nicaraguan citizens. Many of these trained rebels are now cartel officers and leaders. This is one example, among several, of the US interventions in Latin America that have led to increased violence, corruption, and conflict in these countries.[11]

As research on epigenetics continues to demonstrate, experiences of previous generations can have an impact on how genes are expressed in youth today.[12] This contributes to a background framework for understanding risk and resiliency factors of children living in circumstances that lead families to pursue migration. Although most traveling to the United States from Latin America do not meet current qualifications for legal status as refugees, they are frequently survivors of persecution, physical, and sexual abuse.[13] Further, and particularly for those who are entering without authorization, violence is too often a part of the transit process, with detention a possibly distressing end to the journey.[13]

Luis and his family originate from a remote indigenous community in Guatemala, a country with intermittently violent relationships between its government and such communities.

Consideration: How might I be experienced as a representative of a violent authority or, conversely, could this individual be placing complete faith and trust in me as a representative of the nation of refuge and how can I make questioning and disagreement safe for this individual/family?

POSTMIGRATION FACTORS

We also have studies exploring postmigration factors to consider when pursuing health for migrant youth. Borho and colleagues surveyed adolescents with migration backgrounds, and although they were located in Germany, the youth's experiences may be comparable to those in the United States. They found that the most common form of discriminatory behavior experienced was the lack of cultural understanding, followed by social exclusion. Adolescents described experiences of discrimination based on laws such as being unable to obtain a work permit or access health insurance as well as interpersonal discrimination with the example of hearing verbal insults directed their way. Most often youth reported they would respond by leaving the situation, but they also described responding with verbal defenses, boycotting, using deception, resigning, engaging in physical violence, or showing no reaction at all. Youth in this study reported their authority figures, such as teachers, were a critical group who had discriminated against them. Adolescents with darker skin noted additional experiences of discrimination based on this "visible indicator of otherness." Importantly, these youth were able to describe their emotional response related to these experiences, such as anger, aggressiveness, fear, nervousness, acceptance, resignation, helplessness, and astonishment.[14]

These experiences of discrimination impact youth in a myriad of ways. Salas-Wright and colleagues surveyed recently arrived Venezuelan youth aged 10 to 17 year and found that migrant youth who perceived greater levels of discrimination were also more likely to drink alcohol, smoke cigarettes, and use illicit substances.[15] The significance of the impact is even more clear when this is compared with their previous work highlighting that immigrant youth actually tend to use substances at lower rates than their US-born counterparts.[16]

Metzner and colleagues completed a systematic literature review of the impact discrimination had on migrant youth worldwide and found additional concern for effects on self-esteem, interpersonal abilities, lower sense of competence, and lower life satisfaction.[17] Similar findings have been described in other studies along with specific attention given to their negative impact on academic achievement.[18] It is important to highlight that these influences are not inherent in migration alone but have repeatedly been linked to those who experience higher rates of perceived discrimination and trauma along the way.

Another important postmigration form of stress to consider is the discrimination of family members, which leads to direct and indirect effects on children. Alisia G T T Tran's study builds on previous work suggesting that self-perceived experiences of discrimination in parents can negatively impact their children's mental health.[19] In addition to direct discrimination, endorsement of frequently not feeling culturally accepted was associated with poorer parental health and children externalizing and internalizing symptoms.[20]

When Luis first arrived in rural North Carolina, he enrolled in an elementary school with a significant proportion of Latine peers and Spanish speaking staff and was described as highly social and academically engaged. However, when he graduated to middle school, the environment became predominantly non-Hispanic white with only one, noninstructional, staff member identified by the family who they believed could be trusted and with whom they could communicate directly in Spanish.

Consideration: How can my workplace better incentivize diversity in applicants and retained employees? What would help parents feel more culturally celebrated in this space?

Finally, there is an ever-growing body of literature on the acculturation process and acculturative stress in the postmigration period. Lawton and Gerdes provided a definition of acculturation as "changes in the original cultural patterns after direct contact with the host culture group."[21] According to the acculturation model as developed by Berry, these changes typically fit within one of four categories. Using an *integrative* strategy, individuals maintain close relationships with people from their home culture while aspiring to develop relationships with people from the host group. An *assimilative* strategy is used when someone's desire to relate entirely to the host culture leads to rejection of their original culture. On the other end of the spectrum, some will use a *separatist* strategy and reject the host group in favor of a focus on maintaining as much of their own culture as possible. Finally, *marginalization* can occur when individuals are disconnected from both groups and experience ambivalence about cultural connections.[22] Each acculturative approach comes with its own risks and benefits. Overall, strategies that actively engage both cultures are associated with better mental health outcomes, as those who reject either their original or host culture are at an increased risk of impairing acculturative stress.[23]

When families immigrate from Latin America, they may do so as a group, but often it is a process over many years as the family is able to afford the journey for subsequent members. This may provide protective elements as newly arrived individuals are welcomed into family housing and guided to employment and community engagement opportunities. However, tension may develop within families that are at variable stages of, or approaches to, acculturating. Youth in particular may be more quickly immersed in a host culture via school environments and being in earlier developmental stages of identity formation. Family cohesion can suffer even as youth play a critical role in navigating systems of care for less acculturated family members. This is especially true for those immigrating to the United States without a social safety net on arrival. Unstable employment is often associated with a lack of health insurance, long work hours, low wages, and high stress for parents, with children subsequently facing significant unsupervised time, caretaking roles for younger siblings, and pressure to contribute financially.[11] Latine migrant youth are particularly vulnerable to adapting to these pressures through gang involvement with an estimated near 50% of gang members in the United States identifying as Hispanic or Latino and 44% of them being less than the age of 18 year.[24] With gang involved youth experiencing up to 8x the suicide risk relative to non-gang involved youth, a coordinated care response is needed by our systems.[25]

During Luis' illness, his father faced losing his factory job due to missed days of work while visiting his son in the hospital and subsequently the family experienced eviction. Owing to current policies limiting access for unauthorized children to child welfare services, this risked further disenfranchising them from systems of care at a moment of highest need.

Consideration: How can I engage in policy reform focused on enfranchising migrant youth and their families into our communities?

SYSTEMS OF CARE CONSIDERATIONS

As we previously discussed, acculturation is typically defined by the changes that occur within the original culture after coming into contact with the host culture. Although we make no attempt to diminish the importance of continued work to better understand this process and its influences on minoritized individuals, an expanded, more reciprocal view may provide additional pathways to an increasingly equitable future, effective systems, and diminished host–immigrant friction.

In a nation in which access to health care is not guaranteed even for citizens, but education is viewed as a human right, our school systems often become the safety net provider of multiple services. In fact, an estimated 20% of all school-aged children receive some sort of mental health care annually and 60% to 80% of children who receive mental health services do so in the school setting.[26–28] Specifically, unauthorized and asylum-seeking children in the United States have had their right to receive free public education confirmed by the Supreme Court, again reiterating the critical role schools perform in the postmigration process of youth.[29] Teachers, school therapists, nurses, and other staff have anecdotal and formally studied evidence for their direct impact on vulnerable students such as minoritized Latine youth. When youth perceive discrimination by teachers, they are at higher risk of developing depressive symptoms, which are more likely to be expressed as externalizing symptoms than other non-Latine migrant groups.[30–32]

Adapting the acculturation model proposed by Berry, we can assess systems of care according to the approach each is taking when coming into contact with a new culture. In the United States, the term dominant culture is often a pseudonym for White, Western Culture, which has been described as valuing "rugged individualism, competition, action-orientation, hierarchical power structures, standard American English, linear and future time orientation, Judeo-Christianity, European history, Protestant work ethic, objective science, owning goods and property, the nuclear family unit, and European aesthetics."[33] Systems may take a *separatist* approach by requiring migrant youth to assimilate to these values to be included or not provide any pathway for inclusion at all. Liu and colleagues challenged us to consider how the pursuit of assimilating to these values may be a survival strategy of minoritized families that necessarily enacts racial traumas and microaggressions in pursuit of material and psychological safety.[34] Separatist approaches were associated with negative health effects on immigrants and may have detrimental effects on the health of our systems as well.

Once a sufficient enough population shift has taken place, systems may attempt to *assimilate* completely to the new cultural group and reject the original culture. *Marginalization* may occur when ambivalence about change leads to stagnation and disconnection from effective care for any population. Finally, an *integrative* approach seeks to build healthy connections across cultures with value for original ways and openness to new considerations, which is what the remainder of this article will explore. As we consider opportunities for our systems to acculturate in an integrative manner, we must also include the internal work of understanding our own biases and stereotypes so that this work is implemented with a decreased risk of simultaneously enacting microaggressions and racism.[35] Although much more work is needed to better understand how systems can prevent and heal harm enacted during the acculturation process, there is some evidence worth reviewing.

In the current social climate, politicians and media messages may contribute to internalized racism. This is when an individual begins to believe the negative messaging about their group and think less of themselves as a result, possibly encouraging youth to take an assimilationist approach to acculturation.[36] Challenging these messages may begin with personal education on the contributions of Latine communities locally or nationally. For example, to counter messaging that immigrants are taking from limited resources, it could be noted that in 2019 alone, immigrant-led households contributed $330.7 billion in federal taxes and $161.7 billion in combined state and local taxes.[37] As identity development is a major developmental task of adolescence, migrant youth navigating how they will incorporate their ethnicity, nationality, race, sexuality, gender, and so forth may be particularly vulnerable to the effects of negative messaging, especially if it is coming from peers.[38]

Dr Geneva Gay has contributed to our understanding of the capacity teachers have for developing culturally responsive teaching approaches. Her research indicates that creating empathetic relationships and using culturally relevant teaching methods is associated with higher rates of student achievement. Curricula at all levels of education are filled with cultural references, which often come from the dominant culture. Her work challenges educators, be that in the elementary classroom or providing psychoeducation in the clinic, to consider the cultural frame of reference of the learning individual and ensure their frames of reference are included in ways that legitimize their culture and experiences as valid and normal.[39]

Further, cultural values commonly found in Latine households are valuable to actively promote within school and other care settings. One example is familismo, defined as placing a priority not only on the nuclear but also the extended family, which can support the interest of academic, medical, and correctional settings to engage the support system of youth.[40] Incorporating families through communication, volunteering, and decision-making uphold the value of respeto (honoring authority figures) and familismo and have been associated with improvements in academic, social, and emotional well-being.[40] Systems can create motivation for staff to include extended family members when appropriate and should be aware that for some there may be conscious or unconscious resistance, especially if adaptations such as prioritizing the inclusion of a broader family system are seen as more work or challenging their dominant culture congruent values and beliefs.[41]

Working with Luis highlighted that our resident clinic had missed opportunities to intentionally and visibly celebrate the values and cultures of our Latine patients.

Consideration: What languages are present on signage? Are bicultural staff present? What does the decor of the physical space communicate about which cultures are welcome and represented? How are heritage months and religious days of importance celebrated?

The eligibility of migrant youth for any state or federally funded service is a policy question that is thus open for change on all political levels in favor of expanded eligibility regardless of immigration status. However, eligibility alone is not the only barrier. The use of public assistance programs designed to meet the needs of vulnerable children should be explicitly separated from the immigration authorization process of parents to reduce concerns that service access might limit other family members' ability to sponsor or naturalize.[42,43] Awareness raising campaigns may be a useful tool to increase engagement by immigrant parents who are unaware of eligibility or hesitant to accept services for their children due to fears of repercussions given their immigration status.[44] The physical space in which services are rendered provide opportunities for integrative adaptations. As a sense of safety in the use of services increases, the willingness to access services on behalf of their children may also increase. However, additional steps must be taken to assist parents/guardians with system navigation including removing language and literacy barriers.[45]

Consideration: Who is underrepresented in my clinic or classroom? What groups in my area are organizing to expand access to drivers' licenses or pass the Dream Act? What paid opportunities are available for youth after school?

SUMMARY

Migration throughout the Americas is both a historic and current trend with complex factors driving increased movement to the United States and current predictions anticipating only expanding population growth of Hispanic and Latine households in coming years. Expectations that migrant youth bear the full responsibility of adapting to their new surroundings acts to reinforce White and Western supremacy as the only culture with worth and validity.[46] Opportunities exist for individual- and system-level change to better support an integrative process in which our systems not only work more collaboratively but also adapt to ensure culturally appropriate care.

Luis arrived in the United States as a normally developing child but within a couple years, began demonstrating what, in hindsight, can be described as symptoms of acculturation stress. Access to primary health care, mental health care, and welfare services were out of reach for the next 2 years as the school system attempted to fill the gap. Despite their heroic efforts, even this care was impeded by language and trust barriers with social withdrawal and academic decline initially attributed to language deficits instead of to worsening mood and acculturation stress. Although he did not disclose perceived experiences of discrimination, we know this is a common experience for immigrants, and at a minimum, Luis described experiences of being perceived as "different" and was excluded from multiple systems of care based on his immigration status alone. As we learned earlier, attending to the experience of cultural acceptance of the parent may not only directly improve parental mental health but also have indirect positive effects on that of the child and Luis' parents faced safety concerns of immigration and child protective services intervention with each attempt at accessing care. In the end, multiple systems in this rural North Carolina community partnered together to build an effective net of care but it was not until he had endured significant suffering and reached a life-threatening severity of illness.

Luis' story calls on us to take a collaborative systems approach with deliberate efforts to adapt each partner to prioritize inclusion of culturally and linguistically appropriate communication, alignment with the values of youth, diversity of staff, and culturally reflective physical spaces. Further research is needed to better understand the acculturation process of the host culture and the impacts on mental health of various approaches. However, diminishing barriers to accessing services in ways such as expanding use of the preferred language, outreaching communities, and seeking policy protections that expand access are all steps systems of care can begin today in pursuit of healthy futures for Latine migrant youth.

CLINICS CARE POINTS

- Understanding our own stereotypes and biases can help decrease the likelihood we will enact microaggressions on Latine migrant youth.
- When providing education, use culturally relevant frames of reference.
- Normalize cultural values such as familismo as valid through engagement with extended family members when appropriate.
- Pursue the hiring of bilingual and bicultural staff on your team.
- Seek opportunities to highlight the value of the original culture of migrant youth through celebrations of heritage months and religious days.
- Join with local organizations to pursue policy change to expand safe access to systems of care on regional and national levels.

ACKNOWLEDGMENTS

The author would like to thank "Luis" and his family who generously agreed to share their story so that others may learn. Thanks to Sonia Koul (Mountain Area Health Education Center) and Keny Murillo Brizuela (University of North Carolina-Chapel Hill) for their encouragement in pursuing this topic. The author would also like to thank Emily Kulpa (Mountain Area Health Education Center) and Kerry Moreno for their comments on the article.

DISCLOSURE

The author has nothing to disclose.

REFERENCES

1. Virupaksha HG, Kumar A, Nirmala BP. Migration and mental health: an interface. J Nat Sci Biol Med 2014;5(2):233–9.
2. Hirth K, Pillsbury J, Blanton RE. Merchants, markets, and exchange in the Pre-Columbian world. Washington, DC: Dumbarton Oaks Research Library and Collection; 2013.
3. Migration Policy Institute. U.S. immigrant population and share over time, 1850-Present. Available at: https://www.migrationpolicy.org/programs/data-hub/charts/immigrant-population-over-time. Accessed March 23,2023.
4. United States Census Bureau. U.S. census bureau projections show a slower growing, older, more diverse nation a half century from now. 2012. Available at: https://www.census.gov/newsroom/releases/archives/population/cb12-243.html. Accessed March 25, 2023.
5. Child Stats Forum on Child and Family Statistics. 2021. America's children: key national indicators of well-being. 2021. Available at: https://www.childstats.gov/americaschildren21/demo.asp#: ~ :text=This%20population%20is%20projected%20to,1980%20to%2026%25%20in%202020. Accessed March 23, 2023.
6. American Academy of Child & Adolescent Psychiatry. 2023. Systems of care resources. Available at: https://www.aacap.org/AACAP/Practice/Clinical_Practice_Center/Systems_of_Care_and_Collaborative_Models/Systems_of_Care_Resources/AACAP/Clinical_Practice_Center/Systems_of_Care/Resources.aspx?hkey=c3bd9713-878c-4050-b67d-84f51ad68d4d. Accessed August 14, 2023.
7. American Academy of Child & Adolescent Psychiatry. 2023 Collaboration with primary care. Available at: https://www.aacap.org/AACAP/Practice/Clinical_Practice_Center/Systems_of_Care_and_Collaborative_Models/Collaboration_with_Primary_Care/AACAP/Clinical_Practice_Center/Systems_of_Care/Collaboration_with_Primary_Care.aspx?hkey=069b9acd-b629-41fa-8bb8-befe9b1f6387. Accessed August 14, 2023.
8. U.S. Department of Health and Human Resources, Children's Bureau, and Administration for Children and Families. 2023. Mental health and cross-system collaboration. Available at: https://www.childwelfare.gov/topics/systemwide/bhw/collaboration/mh/#: ~ :text=By%20partnering%20across%20systems%2C%20child,development%20and%20mental%20well%2Dbeing. Accessed August 15, 2023.
9. American Academy of Pediatrics. 2023. AAP to create national center for system of services for children with special healthcare needs. Available at: https://www.aap.org/en/news-room/news-releases/aap/2023/aap-to-create-national-center-for-system-of-services-for-children-with-special-health-care-needs/. Accessed August 15, 2023.
10. Skidmore TE, Smith PH, Green JN. Colonial foundations. In: *Modern Latin America*. 8th edition. New York: Oxford University Press; 2012. p. 18–111.
11. National Hispanic and Latino MHTTC. Latino youth gangs prevention in the school system. 2023. Available at: https://mhttcnetwork.org/centers/national-hispanic-and-latino-mhttc/product/latino-youth-gangs-prevention-school-system. Accessed April 4, 2023.
12. Collins N, Roth T. Intergenerational transmission of stress-related epigenetic regulation. Developmental Human Behavioral Epigenetics 2021;23:119–41.

13. Sangalang CC, Becerra D, Mitchell FM, et al. Trauma, post-migration stress, and mental health: a comparative analysis of refugees and immigrants in the United States. J Immigr Minor Health 2019;21:909–19.
14. Borho A, Morawa E, Schug C, et al. Perceived post-migration discrimination: the perspective of adolescents with migration background. Eur Child Adolesc Psychiatry 2022.
15. Salas-Wright CP, Schwartz SJ, Cohen M, et al. Cultural stress and substance use risk among Venezuelan migrant youth in the United States. Subst Use Misuse 2020;55(13):2175–83.
16. Salas-Wright CP, Vaughn MG, Schwartz SJ, et al. An "immigrant paradox" for adolescent externalizing behavior? Evidence from a national sample. Soc Psychiatr Psychiatr Epidemiol 2016;51(1):27–37.
17. Metzner F, Adedeji A, Wichmann MLY, et al. Experiences of discrimination and everyday racism among children and adolescents with an immigrant background - results of a systematic literature review on the impact of discrimination on the developmental outcomes of minors worldwide. Front Psychol 2022;13:805941.
18. Benner AD, Wang Y, Shen Y, et al. Racial/ethnic discrimination and well-being during adolescence: a meta-analytic review. Am Psychol 2018;73(7):55–83.
19. Tran AGTT. Family contexts: parental experiences of discrimination and child mental health. Am J Community Psychol 2014;53(1–2):37–46.
20. Tran AG. Family contexts: parental experiences of discrimination and child mental health. Am J Community Psychol 2014;53(1):37–46.
21. Lawton KE, Gerdes AC. Acculturation and Latino adolescent mental health: integration of individual, environmental, and family influences. Clin Child Fam Psychol Rev 2014;17:385–98.
22. Berry JW, Kim U, Power S, et al. Acculturation attitudes in plural societies. Appl Psychol 1989;38(2):185–206.
23. Urzúa A, Ferrer R, Canales Gaete V, et al. The influence of acculturation strategies in quality of life by immigrants in Northern Chile. Qual Life Res 2017;26(3):717–26.
24. National Gang Intelligence Center. National youth gang survey analysis: demographics. Available at: https://nationalgangcenter.ojp.gov/survey-analysis/demographics#anchorregm. Accessed March 25, 2023.
25. Coid JW, Ullrich S, Keers R, et al. Gang membership, violence, and psychiatric morbidity. Am J Psychiatr 2013;170(9):985–93.
26. Foster S, Rollefson M, et al. School Mental Health Services in The United States, 2002-2003. Substance Abuse and Mental Health Services Administration. 2005. Available at: https://eric.ed.gov/?id=ED499056 Accessed March 25, 2023.
27. Green JG, McLaughlin KA, Alegría M, et al. School mental health resources and adolescent mental health service use. J Am Acad Child Adolesc Psychiatry 2013;52(5):501–10.
28. Patel SG, Bouche V, Thomas I, et al. Mental health and adaptation among newcomer immigrant youth in United States educational settings. Curr Opin Psychol 2023;49:101459.
29. Pyler v. Doe, 457 US 202. (1982).
30. Lopez WD, LeBrón AM, Graham LF, et al. Discrimination and depressive symptoms among Latina/o adolescents of immigrant parents. Int Q Community Health Educ 2016;36(2):131–40.
31. Kim J, Nicodimos S, Kushner SE, et al. Comparing mental health of US children of immigrants and non-immigrants in 4 racial/ethnic groups. J Sch Health 2018;88(2):167–75.

32. Céspedes YM, Huey SJ Jr. Depression in Latino adolescents: a cultural discrepancy perspective. Cult Divers Ethnic Minor Psychol 2008;14(2):168–72.
33. Katz JH. The sociopolitical nature of counseling. Counsel Psychol 1985;13(4): 615–24.
34. Liu MW, Liu RZ, Garrison YL, et al. Racial trauma, microaggressions, and becoming racially innocuous: the role of acculturation and white supremacist ideology. Am Psychol 2019;74(1):143–55.
35. Sue DW, Capodilupo CM, Torino GC, et al. Racial microaggressions in everyday life: implications for clinical practice. Am Psychol 2007;62(4):271–86.
36. Jones CP. Levels of racism: a theoretic framework and a gardener's tale. Am J Public Health 2000;90(8):1212–5.
37. American Immigration Council. Immigrants in the United States. 2021. Available at: https://www.americanimmigrationcouncil.org/research/immigrants-in-the-united-states. Accessed March 23, 2023.
38. Wahlstrom D, White T, Luciana M. Neurobehavioral evidence for changes in dopamine system activity during adolescence. Neurosci Biobehav Rev 2010; 34(5):631–48.
39. Gay G. Ethnic and cultural diversity in curriculum content. In: Culturally responsive teaching: theory, research and practice. 3rd edition. New York: Teachers College Press; 2018. p. 142–96.
40. Maiya S, Carlo G, Gülseven Z, et al. Direct and indirect effects of parental involvement, deviant peer affiliation, and school connectedness on prosocial behaviors in U.S. Latino/a youth. J Soc Pers Relationships 2020;37(10–11):2898–917.
41. DiAngelo R. White fragility. Int Nat J Critical Pedagogy 2011;3:54–70.
42. Perreira K M, Crosnoe R, et al. Barriers to immigrants' access to health and human services programs. 2012. Available at: https://aspe.hhs.gov/reports/barriers-immigrants-access-health-human-services-programs-0. Accessed March 25, 2023.
43. American Immigration Council. 2021. Why don't immigrants apply for citizenship? Available at: https://www.americanimmigrationcouncil.org/sites/default/files/research/why_dont_immigrants_apply_for_citizenship_0.pdf. Accessed March 23, 2023.
44. Alvira-Hammond M, Gennetian L. How Hispanic parents perceive their need and eligibility for public assistance. 2012. Available at: https://hispanicrescen.wpengine.com/wp-content/uploads/2015/12/2015-46Hisp-Ctr-Perceptions-Eligibility.pdf Accessed April 4, 2023.
45. Karina F, Chaudry A. 2011. A comprehensive review of immigrant access to health and human services. The Urban Institute. Available at: https://www.urban.org/sites/default/files/publication/27651/412425-A-Comprehensive-Review-of-Immigrant-Access-to-Health-and-Human-Services.PDF. Accessed April 4, 2023.
46. Holoien DS, Shelton JN. You deplete me: the cognitive costs of colorblindness on ethnic minorities. J Exp Soc Psychol 2012;48(2):562–5.

Worcester Refugee Assistance Project

An Example of Strengths-Based, Community-Based, Culturally Sensitive Care

Emily Hochstetler, MD[a],*, Omar Taweh, BS, BA[a,1],
Anushay J. Mistry, MD[b,2], Peter Metz, MD[a,3]

KEYWORDS

- Refugee • Immigrant • Community • Mental health • System of Care
- Strengths-based care

KEY POINTS

- The needs of refugee youth are unique and involve considerations of culture, religion, family structure, and personal life experiences.
- Mental health care priorities may be different for refugee populations for a variety of reasons and may need to be structured more informally—focusing on building community supports and creating a place of nonjudgment is key.
- Providing holistic care for the family is often one of the best ways to support refugee youth.
- System of Care principles should be used as a framework when conceptualizing approaches to these populations.

INTRODUCTION

Given the increase in the number of migrants in the United States over the last two decades,[1] it is of increasing importance to learn how to address the needs of youth from different cultures and backgrounds. Along with an increased number of migrants has been an increase in the number of research studies focused on refugees' mental health. Numerous studies looking at the psychological effects of adverse childhood experiences associated with resettlement have shown a higher prevalence of

[a] University of Massachusetts, T.H. Chan School of Medicine, 55 Lake Avenue North, Worcester, MA 01655, USA; [b] Children's Hospital Los Angeles, 4650 Sunset Boulevard, Los Angeles, CA 90027, USA
[1] ,Present address: 55 N Lake Avenue, Worcester, MA, 01605
[2] Present address: 21 Oakley Lane, Waltham, MA 02452, USA
[3] PO Box 166, West, Stockbridge, MA 01266, USA
* Corresponding author. 55 N Lake Avenue, Worcester, MA 01605.
E-mail address: emily.hochstetler@gmail.com

Child Adolesc Psychiatric Clin N Am 33 (2024) 263–276
https://doi.org/10.1016/j.chc.2023.10.003
1056-4993/24/© 2023 Elsevier Inc. All rights reserved.

post-traumatic stress disorder as well as both internalizing and externalizing problems.[2] However, there is still a dearth of research into the socioemotional needs of refugee children and how to meet these needs.[3] One of the challenges of this area of research is a significant variation in the obstacles facing refugees due to the immense variability in the circumstances leading to the need for resettlement.[4] There can be any number of stressors in the preflight, flight, and resettlement periods, in addition to the stresses of being in new surroundings, with different cultural norms and expectations.[5] This leads to the necessity for careful tailoring of support programs to meet each child's individual needs.

The purpose of this article is to present an example of an organization, the Worcester Refugee Assistance Project (WRAP), which provides care to refugees in the community and discusses their services through the lens of the System of Care (SOC) framework. WRAP is known in the community as an institution that strives to provide quality support to migrants and refugees, and though it was not founded with explicit SOC values in mind, when the services that they provide are examined one can see multiple SOC values and principles exhibited, which contribute to the success that they have had in providing services to these populations. Examining the ways in which these values are enacted is helpful when considering the creation of similar organizations. In addition, this article aims to demonstrate the ways in which strengths-based and culturally competent care can be practically enacted, as well as the challenges that can be encountered during implementation of this approach. For refugee youth, the application of these concepts is especially important and challenging. The authors specifically discuss the core SOC concepts of family-driven and youth-guided, community-based care, cultural competency, strengths-based care, prevention/early intervention, individualized services, and transition-age supports. The authors focus on how these concepts have been used and the challenges that have been faced, incorporating real-life feedback from the people involved in these programs.

WORCESTER REFUGEE ASSISTANCE PROJECT
Background

The WRAP is an independent 501(c) (3) nonprofit organization dedicated to the empowerment of local refugees, primarily from Myanmar and Afghanistan, toward sustainable self-reliance through advocacy, educational support, and mentoring. Originally founded in 2009 by a nursing student at the University of Massachusetts Chan Medical School, the primary goal of WRAP was to assist the growing local Burmese community in achieving financial independence, establishing a community across multicultural backgrounds, and learning how to navigate the local resources necessary to succeed in their new home. For the past 12 years, WRAP has collaborated with other local organizations both in Worcester and the Greater Boston area to assist Burmese refugees and more recently Afghan refugees, with the challenges of resettlement and to create programming to assist with children, youth, and adult personal and professional development.

Owing to their status as newly resettled refugees, corresponding socioeconomic backgrounds, and developing English proficiency, the population that WRAP serves is particularly vulnerable to xenophobia and racial discrimination. Refugee youth are coming of age in a particularly racially charged environment where immigration is an increasingly polarizing topic and where immigrant families around the country are facing state-based persecution and antipathy. The immigrant experience has been reduced in the public sphere to simple numbers and questions of legality as opposed to compassionate support and guidance. These challenges have led WRAP to create programming to help children and youth develop positive coping mechanisms through wellness and mindfulness in the face of adversity.

Programming

One example of such programming is the WRAP Mentoring Project, a project started by medical students at the University of Massachusetts Chan Medical School geared toward creating positive relationships between mentors and WRAP children and youth, specifically children aged 4 to 13 year and youth 14 to 21 year. Students from the University of Massachusetts Chan Medical School are paired with a refugee youth or child to provide emotional support, friendship, and guidance; to date, more than 30 pairings have been made. Most of the youth who participate in WRAP have seen or personally experienced significant traumas in their lives, yet have never before had the opportunity to process their traumas in a facilitated environment. These youth have demonstrated truly remarkable resilience and through the WRAP programming are offered support within their community in dealing with their past trauma while also navigating the unique difficulties of moving to a new country and adjusting to a new culture. The selection of mentor–mentee pairing is tailored to the needs of the youth and children, as well as the skills and availability of the mentor. Mentor–mentee pairings meet weekly or biweekly and engage in activities jointly agreed on that are either social or educational, and weekly feedback is collected from mentors regarding their relationship and discussions with their mentees. Mentors and those running various groups are composed primarily of UMass Chan Medical students, Clark University undergraduate students, and other members of the Worcester community. In addition to providing services for the youth served, this program also encourages the development of cultural humility within the mentors.

Other examples of past youth programming include the 2016 book publication titled *When We Were Home* and the Making Worcester Home initiative in association with Worcester State University. *When We Were Home* was a compilation of drawings from WRAP youth depicting their personal experiences both in their homelands and as newly arrived refugees in Worcester. The Making Worcester Home Project earned youth one college course credit and allowed youth to design and analyze an issue of their choosing in the Worcester area.

Collaborations

WRAP works extensively with the many refugee and migrant advocacy organizations in Worcester, MA (**Fig. 1**). It is a member of the Worcester Together Refugee Response, a citywide partnership initially formed to address and support the city's response to COVID-19s impact on migrants. WRAP collaborates with many local organizations to support resettled people toward self-reliance through mentoring, advocacy, and educational assistance.

Examples include Tower Hill Botanic Garden and the Burncoat Center for Crafts, which provide opportunities for youth and children to participate in educational and age-appropriate activities. Along with local religious organizations such as the Worcester Islamic Center and Welcoming Alliance for Refugee Ministry, WRAP helps facilitate access to culturally appropriate community support. WRAP also engages in bilateral collaboration with local advocacy organizations such as United Way and other community grant groups with funding programming for its children/youth/education groups—more than 50,000 dollars have been awarded to the organization in 2023 alone to fund educational opportunities for our growing youth and children groups. WRAP works with local universities to provide opportunities for passionate students

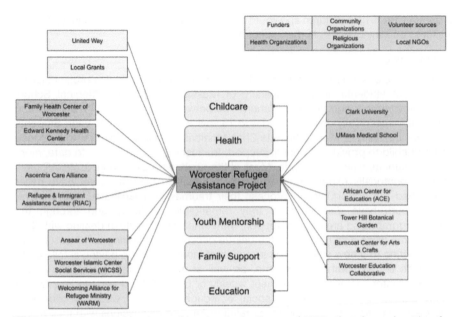

Fig. 1. WRAP is proximal to several local organizations and NGOs that do work with refugees and migrants. WRAP is developed and funded by volunteers coming from schools and local donor groups.

to become involved with supporting the education of refugees from the primary school to collegiate level that include, but are not limited to, education, programming, health care delivery, and grassroots organizing. Most importantly, volunteers of WRAP often serve as mediators of dialogue between large organizations that operate independently to help consolidate efforts and resources to better deliver support to migrant and refugee youth and children.

WRAPs work supporting refugees in the Worcester area is done by volunteers coming from the UMass Chan Medical School, Clark University, and other local Non Governmental Organizations (NGOs), which provides it with the unique ability to connect community organizations through students.

SYSTEM OF CARE FRAMEWORK

The SOC approach was initiated in the 1980s by the National Institute of Mental Health and subsequently through the federal Substance Abuse and Mental Health Services Administration. It has evolved over time and is now the standard framework to support the expansion and transformation of supports and services for youth with behavioral health needs and their families within public child serving agencies and organizations at the federal level as well as the state and county level in most states. The values and principles of the SOC approach include that care must be family-driven and youth-guided—meaning that the person(s) served have voice and choice to identify and prioritize their needs in the overarching effort to achieve well-being for the child and family. These values also include community-based and culturally competent care that rests on the principles of a complete biopsychosocial assessment; strengths-based, individualized, and trauma-informed care; continuity of care across transitions; and prevention, early intervention, and resilience, among others.[6] Many of these concepts overlap and interconnect, which means that one service can incorporate multiple concepts and serve multiple different needs.

SYSTEM OF CARE FRAMEWORK AT WORCESTER REFUGEE ASSISTANCE PROJECT

The SOC framework is a useful way to analyze the success of WRAP within the Worcester community. SOC core principles are flexible, can be applied across multiple settings, and seem differently depending on the ways in which they are applied in different situations. Below, the authors first discuss salient SOC concepts, and then how they have been used, informally or not, at WRAP, as well as the challenges that have been faced in their implementation. Please reference **Table 1** for specific quotes pulled from the WRAP mentoring program categorized by the SOC concept that they exemplify. These quotes come directly and with consent from weekly "check-in" journals of mentors involved in the WRAP Mentoring Program.

System of Care Concept 1: Family-Driven and Youth-Guided

The supports and services provided by WRAP grew directly out of the self-identified needs of the population served—Burmese and Afghan refugees resettled in Worcester, MA. WRAP collaborates with organizations that provide federally funded resettlement support, such as Ascentria Care Alliance and the Refugee & Immigrant Assistance Center, to identify and remedy the unmet needs of resettled people.

In addition to the WRAP youth mentorship program discussed above, WRAP runs a care navigation program where case managers from the Worcester Free Care Collaborative—free clinics in the Worcester area run by UMass Medical School graduate Students—connect families and youth with higher level resources that they may be experiencing difficulty in accessing. Examples of resources that the care navigation program connects families with include, but are not limited to, enrollment of children for school, applying for food stamps, and enrollment in MassHealth insurance.

WRAP addresses gaps in community education needs by hosting weekly sessions where older community members come together to receive teaching regarding a broad range of self-selected topics such as COVID-19, applying for jobs, and accessing transportation services. Childcare is provided to adult members to allow for an opportunity to socialize and learn without worry for children. Education is delivered by local WRAP volunteers as well as local undergraduate and graduate students. In addition, WRAP has unofficial adult mentorship that more closely resembles friendship with adult community members.

System of Care Concept 2: Cultural Competency

Cultural competency within an SOC framework focuses on the importance of care being delivered within the context of the patient's culture, and the difference this can make in how care is received. The importance of this concept cannot be overstated, as many of the criteria which mental health services identify as needing treatment may not be considered problematic or abnormal in different cultures.[7] This concept overlaps with the core concept of individualized services and can also overlap with strengths-based care, as in many cases cultural values can enhance treatment when properly used.

WRAP strives to exemplify cultural humility in the Worcester community through such programming as the Mentoring Program at UMass Chan Medical School, where the mentees are both mentored and shared their lived experiences with their mentors, future health care professionals. Through this model, the program is able to simultaneously serve the needs of the refugees and augment the training of medical

Table 1
A weekly mentor check-in via google form posed focused questions to mentors regarding mentor–mentee activities and relationships, as well as mentee behaviors, safety, family and home life, and education

Theme#	Theme	Sample Quotes
1	Family-Driven and Youth-Guided	Quote 1A: "really likes watching anime movies. We watched an anime movie showing while his parents were out applying jobs." Quote 1B: "We have talked about applying to colleges together, which her family does not know much about. She's been asking questions about the process of applying and what life as a college student looks like. We have been able to bond over our discussions about college applications."
2	Cultural Competency	Quote 2A: "does not feel like a mentor-mentee relationship. More akin to friendship. Mentee seems mature, pursing electrical engineering with clear, and concrete goals. We share a commonality where our parents are immigrants. In our last meeting, we discussed similar experiences we had growing up with such a background. Another unrelated but shared experience between us is being raised Catholic and serving as alter servers when we were younger." Quote 2B: "We discussed our shared interest in Kpop and our similar intra-family relationships. She is excited about going to college to learn about herself, and we talked about how I navigated that experience with immigrant parents as well."
3	Community-Based Treatment	Quote 3A: "We attended the Burncoat Festival with her family, and interacted with some of the local community organizations doing education and activities for young people. We walked around with her parents and had Burmese food"
4	Strengths-Based Care	Quote 4A: "He seems comfortable talking/venting about school and work. He's leaning toward pre-med and sometimes it is a bit difficult for myself, as a medical student, to judge how involved I should be in terms of academics, He does appreciate and value our discussions regarding medicine." Quote 4B: "I was really impressed with his reading. There were a number of words that he picked up easily, and can read most basic words (even if some take prompting and sounding out letter by letter). I was really excited to see that."
5	Prevention and Early Intervention	Quote 5A: "He did mention a few things about the COVID vaccine that I tried to probe as much as I could without overstepping. He said that neither of his parents are vaccinated and though he initially was hesitant about getting the vaccine, he is considering doing it soon." Quote 5B: "We reviewed department of transitional assistance benefits and practicing using an ATM machine to prepare her for being an adult."

(continued on next page)

| **Table 1** | | |
| **(continued)** | | |
Theme#	Theme	Sample Quotes
6	Individualized Services	Quote 6A: "It is noticeable how tired he is each week (yawning, putting his head down in front of the camera, etc). He told me that he wakes up before 7, so by the time our session comes around, he's been doing school/work related activities for a big chunk of the day. I'm thinking of proposing 5 PM instead in case that's better for him." Quote 6B: "We also worked on conversation practice through the phone as she expressed that she wants to become less shy and be able to talk more with new people. We ended our phone-call by sharing our 3 happy moments of the week."
7	Transition-Age Supports	Quote 7A: "He opened up about his family's current housing struggles with me." Quote 7B: "When he was talking about school he was also talking about how he just feels tired. I tried to express to him that if he needs anything that I was there for him and to try and stay positive during trying times like this. Moments like this aren't very typical with him and it was one of the few times that the has ever talked to me about times that he struggling with things."

Selected quotes are organized by the System of Care concept that they represent.

personnel.[8] This enhances the health care training of the mentors, allowing them to be more aware of the importance of being a physician with cultural humility and the nuances of providing care to patients from diverse backgrounds.[9]

One challenge that the WRAP executive board has faced consistently throughout the years has been the difficulty of ensuring a sufficient number of board members with lived experiences of being a refugee and resettling in a new country. Despite a large number of adults in the community WRAP serves, most of these refugees are focused, by necessity, on supporting their families, and achieving economic stability; refugee community members have vocalized their concern that at times, board membership has made it difficult for them to commit to serve on the WRAP executive board due to a lack of time and energy. As a result, key perspectives from the community being served have at times been underrepresented in discussions regarding WRAPs programming. However, the addition of community members on our community board has allowed us to better assess the impact of our programs and services provided to more than 60 kids in our youth and children's group.

System of Care Concept 3: Community-Based Treatment

Community-based treatment is the practice of using preexisting and newly created community structures to enhance access to services ranging from childcare to health care. The advantages of community-based care are broad and include service delivery by people with nuanced knowledge about local infrastructure, local and easy accessibility of supports and services for communities served, and flexible models of support that can be adapted and modified on an as-needed basis and that avoid the disruption of the family and community that services provided outside of the community cause.[10] In many ways, within the refugee communities, this SOC concept overlaps with strengths-based care (discussed below), as one of the most noticeable strengths within the refugee population is the focus on family and community bonds. The current research concerning community-based care in refugee communities is lacking and faces many challenges.[11]

Historically, the response to a western approach to mental health care within the refugee population has varied widely due to complex and nuanced psychosocial factors including, but not limited to, the stigmatization of receiving mental health treatment in many cultures. Because of this, it is important to be able to integrate protective services within the community, where people feel safe to seek support and help. In some cases, this means the leveraging of community members as agents of facilitating mental health care while also providing alternative options to those who may deliberately choose to obtain it outside of their community. In this way, community-based care and cultural competency are inherently linked, as in many cases (and especially in migrant and refugee populations) supports and services may be better received when provided within the context of a community where these populations already feel connected. WRAP does not provide explicit mental health care services, rather embracing and encouraging the ways in which mental health care can be promoted in an informal context.

WRAP has developed and facilitated several programs with and for the local Burmese and Afghan refugee communities. They work to connect newly resettled Afghan youth and children with similarly aged Burmese kids through weekly education sessions, opportunities for peer mentoring, and regularly scheduled opportunities for entire family unit engagement, all within a short distance from family homes. Strengths in this approach include the extensive relationship between WRAP volunteers and the Burmese community, which translate to trust building between the two communities and the Afghan community with WRAP. By facilitating relationship building through active community integration efforts and programming, WRAP takes an advantage of both previous advocacy work the organization had done, inherent diversity of the Worcester community, and commonly shared experiences to support youth. These programs actively build on the community supports that are naturally present, to create a new network of support.

One of the challenges in the implementation of this concept is directly related to one of its strengths: WRAPs mission is accomplished by the intrinsic motivation of volunteers to support refugee youth. This makes volunteers passionate, but also more likely to feel less responsibility to the organization. Relying heavily on both graduate and undergraduate students to create and implement programming for refugee youth creates a direct connection to grassroots developed resources and knowledge but also makes programming heavily subject to the direct influence of student availability amid variable academic calendars.

System of Care Concept 4: Strengths-Based Care

Strengths-based care departs from the historically "problem-focused" treatment of the past and moves into care based on using the strengths of the adolescents served to reach their goals. This moves from an approach that often engenders shame (ie, "There is something wrong with me") to one that encourages hope via focus on current skills and areas of strength. This encourages both providers and persons served to focus on current resources that the person has, whether those are internal (Are they really good at art? Languages? Do they have a remarkable amount of resilience? Kindness?) or external (Do they have family support? Friend support? Live in a community with resources?). Doing so enables the better use of these strengths in healing. In evidence of this, implementation of strengths-based care on one child and adolescent inpatient unit resulted in a 75% reduction in total hours of seclusion and restraint over the course of 1 year.[12] Further research is indicated on the impacts of strengths-based care in a community setting. However, anecdotally this has been helpful (as described below).

Although strengths-based care is harder to implement individually with the WRAP children's group due to the quantity of children participating, elements of strengths-based care are inherent in the structure of the group. Based on the availability of volunteers, they often divide children into groups, such as level of language proficiency or previously identified academic strengths, and provide play or education catered to the subgroup of children's specific needs to encourage growth in these areas of identified strengths. This helps to build confidence within the children involved. In addition, the children's mentoring program pairs local graduate and undergraduate students with one or two kids and allows them to engage in regular reading, math, or writing practice, targeted to their specific needs and strengths. Through WRAPs youth mentoring program, local graduate students create direct and personal relationships with participants and support them to reach their academic, personal, technical, or artistic goals using grant funding. Older youth are actively involved in choosing the types of programs planned for them (via monitored group chats), for example, going indoor rock climbing, art therapy sessions, or having a movie night, which gives them more agency in deciding how they would like to spend their time. Through involvement in the Mentoring Program, youth have been able to receive support in reaching their goals and growing their strengths.

System of Care Concept 5: Prevention/Early Intervention

Prevention and early intervention focuses on the idea that if healthy services and supports can be implemented earlier in a person's life trajectory, then many of the difficulties that may be faced later in life will be significantly mitigated or avoided altogether. Prevention and early intervention often overlap, as many people who engage in preventative services may already be at the stage of needing early intervention. It is also important to note that prevention/early intervention does not refer to a single approach or way of doing things: "Primary prevention is not a single uniform strategy that achieves uniform results, but a collection of distinct approaches that are likely to vary in outcome depending on the level of intervention, target population, program objectives, and specific circumstances of the intervention."[13] In this way, the core concept of prevention/early intervention also overlaps with the concept of individualization of services. It is important to keep in mind how services focused around prevention/early intervention will be received in the communities served, and so by necessity in the migrant and refugee populations these services may look different than those in the population at large. Providing programming to support and strengthen the family itself allows for earlier and more sustainable preventative measures due to the individualized tailoring of programming according to community input.[14]

By connecting the WRAP children and youth both with each other and the community at large, WRAP plays a large role in providing opportunities for children and youth to interact with adults outside their home. Through these opportunities, WRAP programming serves as a first-line defense against the inherent mental struggles associated with acclimating to a new country, culture, and experiences. One of the strengths of the WRAP model of programming is the focus on the whole family: "Preventive mental health interventions that aim to stop, lessen, or delay possible negative individual mental health and behavioral sequelae through improving family and community protective resources in resettled refugee families are needed."[15] WRAP provides focused programming for children, adolescents, and adults, allowing for holistic care of each family member. In this way, every family member is provided with support both from their community itself and other adults in the surrounding community. This approach highlights strengths-based care, focusing on the strengths of the families involved and how WRAP can augment those strengths to prevent or allow for early interventions on the mental health challenges facing refugee populations.

System of Care Concept 6: Individualized Services

The concept of individualized services integrates many of the values discussed above. For example, individualization of treatment can involve identifying the individual's strengths, community supports, and possibly unique cultural supports. Much of mental health treatment, by necessity, begins as formulaic. However, when this formulaic basis is then applied and transformed to an individualized care plan, the care has the potential to become significantly more effective, both because the person can be more fully seen and heard, and also because they can be more involved in creating the plan themselves and thereby building agency. Family-driven and youth-guided care inherently supports individualized care. As has been discussed above, migrant and refugee youth are at especially high risk, making the benefit of person-centered individualized services clear. One of the main challenges associated with the provision of mental health care to refugee populations is the underestimation of the prevalence and severity of the mental health needs of refugees.[16] Insufficient attention is often paid to the variability of trauma symptoms due to cultural insensitivity and hesitations to self-report. Further exacerbating the difficulty of identifying mental health challenges in refugee populations is the complex nature of the trauma sequelae on cross-cultural child development.

Refugee children and youth exist at different stages of maturity, development, and growth, often independent of their peers or age. Each one requires support and services that look different than those for others based on a number of different variables that include learning style, personality type, and previous experiences including traumas. WRAP uses active mechanisms improvement of programs such as feedback forms while delivering support to more than 60 Afghan and Burmese refugee families in the Greater Worcester area, each of which have notably different needs, strengths, and weaknesses in caring for youth and children during development. Afghan families ask for (and receive) support understanding how to use emergency rooms and primary care offices, whereas Burmese families ask for (and receive) assistance planning for sending youth to college and other institutions of higher education. These individualized services are delivered to the different groups that WRAP serves, in part due to differences in years since resettlement but also due to specific requests from community members. WRAP also individualizes the relationships between mentors and mentees in its youth and children's mentoring groups. Mentors in the children's program work with families to provide mentorship that can make family life easier or that focus on experiences the child is struggling with understanding. Mentors in the youth program identify interests held by different subgroups of the youth group—such as art, outdoors activities, and movies—and plan opportunities for relationship building with them in mind. Intentional pairing of mentors and mentees with similar interests or life experiences strengthens the impact of the support provided to the youth and children.

System of Care Concept 7: Transition-Age Supports

Periods of transitions are a time when people are particularly in need of additional support due to increased vulnerability during acquisition of new responsibilities and formation of behavior patterns. In addition, refugee youth often experience different types of transition periods at different times due to the cultural differences, family needs and expectations, and social maturity. Given the broad variability in maturity among youth with different experiences is important for programs to be flexible with age-specific services. However, despite these differences, most of support programs focus on the transition period from high school to college, thus excluding refugee youth who do not attend college. A search for ("transition-age" AND "refugee") and other variations on this on PubMed yielded zero results, demonstrating the need for further research into the needs of transition-age youth in the refugee population.

In order to support refugee youth through the period of transition from high school to the next stage of their lives, one program that WRAP offers is college preparatory services to augment the Youth and Mentoring programs. These services assist college-aged youth with the college application process and with scholarship assistance. As part of this program, WRAP also hosts bi-monthly discussion groups for young adults of various high school ages to share their experiences and struggles with their peers as well as mentors for advice, guidance, and support. In addition, a major challenge for WRAP youth who seek to further educate themselves is balancing their familial responsibilities. In many Asian cultures, it is the responsibility of the youth to care for the family once they reach young adulthood.[17] Youth who seek to leave the household, for example, to pursue further education, are at times, expected to balance caring for the family with pursuing their academic or professional goals. The dissonance between family responsibility and personal aspiration has often been a source of contention for youth supported by WRAP. As these expectations often hinder youth's attempts to pursue other opportunities, WRAP also supports youth during this transition period by helping families find other avenues of support such as childcare, timely education, and monetary assistance.

FURTHER CHALLENGES

Since its inception, WRAP has maintained a high level of flexibility in working with changing populations, variable resources, and fluctuating levels of public support. Although WRAPs work fills a number of gaps in care provided to refugee communities in Worcester, MA, there are limitations to its work and challenges that it is not always best equipped to navigate.

As with any nonprofit organization, turnover of volunteers is always a concern. Specifically for WRAP, its origin as an organization run by nursing and medical students in the middle of intense health care degree granting programs has created a number of roadblocks in creating a consistent volunteer pool with whom refugee youth are able to create trusting relationships. The development of the WRAP mentorship program, where youth are paired one-on-one with a student mentor, addressed this gap, facilitating relationships that were lower intensity but more consistent. The mentoring program, however, is imperfect due to the fact that student mentors in health care degree programs have demanding schedules, sometimes with minimal time available for extracurricular involvement. Expansion of the program to undergraduate students is in development and will hopefully provide somewhat of a more consistent mentor–mentee dynamic over the course of 4 years.

Integration of youth group members into the local community is a goal of WRAP. The organization has been successful in supporting students to become involved locally in a number of capacities including sports, technology, and art. However, there is the challenge of integration into local communities due to cultural, language, and social barriers. WRAP youth—with Burmese and Afghan background—join the Worcester ecosystem with inherent differences that separate them from their peers. Focused efforts by local school systems, in conjunction with local refugee advocacy organizations, have proven to be successful in addressing some, but not all, of the barriers that limit refugee youth from becoming integrated within their communities.

WRAP is one of a broad number of local organizations and institutions that aims to provide direct support to refugee and migrant families in the Worcester area. As is with most nonprofit and humanitarian work, less than optimal communication between agencies with similar goals can create challenges for organizers. With the influx of Afghan migrants to Worcester, the leaders of these organizations came together to strategize support for the new community members. Coalitions, like the Worcester Together group facilitated by the city, have made significant strides in limiting the duplication of efforts, building out collaboration between groups with different skill sets, and aiding in appropriate distribution of federal funding among groups. This effort is consistent with the core SOC concept of care coordination.

Another concern is that, like many other cities in the United States, Worcester is currently experiencing a rapid gentrification of its neighborhoods. Refugee families that were originally able to remain financially afloat and provide their families the resources needed to thrive are now navigating higher costs secondary to both inflation and gentrification and being displaced to the surrounding towns. Several city-wide programs, WRAP, and other nonprofit programs have been developed to provide food, clothing, and childcare assistance to families, with high levels of success.

SUMMARY

When considering the needs of refugee and migrant youth, there are a multitude of factors to consider. The authors have touched on a few of these here, especially regarding building an organization that prioritizes these needs. Through the groups and mentoring that recognize the needs and strengths of refugees from childhood through to young adulthood, WRAP has been able to reach hundreds of at-risk youth over the past 10 years, with numbers of kids in the children's and youth group fluctuating between 40 and 60 in any given school year or summer.

Creating an organization that integrates SOC values can be challenging; however, the support and care offered can be incredibly impactful. We encourage anyone hoping to build an organization that offers care to migrants and refugees to consider these SOC values as they provide care to these populations.

ACKNOWLEDGMENTS

We thank Nathan Yingling (University of Massachusetts Chan Medical School) for being a driving force for the collection of feedback regarding youth and children experiences with WRAP. This article was significantly strengthened with his work, and additionally the work of the countless UMass Chan medical student volunteers that mentored and supported the young people of the WRAP community. We thank Vanessa Avalone, Meme Tran, MD, Millie Rao, and countless others of the WRAP leadership for their advocacy for the children that they serve.

CLINICS CARE POINTS

- Refugee and migrant populations face unique challenges, and often a traditional Western behavioral health approach may not be effective for a variety of reasons. It is useful to focus on building community supports and providing places of acceptance and nonjudgment.

- SOC) values and principles provide assistance in developing sensitive, strengths-based approaches.
- A single service can incorporate multiple SOC concepts.
- It can be difficult to engage migrants or refugees with lived experience in full-time positions in an organization due to lack of availability. In these cases, it is best to involve them in whatever ways work best for their lives and schedules and maintain an open and consistent route of communication for feedback.

DISCLOSURE

None of the authors have conflicts to disclose.

REFERENCES

1. Ward N, Batalova J. Frequently Requested Statistics on Immigrants and Immigration in the United States. migrationpolicy.org. Published March 17, 2022. https://www.migrationpolicy.org/article/frequently-requested-statistics-immigrants-and-immigration-united-states
2. Khan NZ, Shilpi AB, Sultana R, et al. Displaced Rohingya children at high risk for mental health problems: Findings from refugee camps within Bangladesh. Child Care Health Dev 2018;45(1):28–35.
3. Bronstein I, Montgomery P. Psychological distress in refugee children: a systematic review. Clin Child Fam Psychol Rev 2011;14(1):44–56.
4. Nakeyar C, Esses V, Reid GJ. The psychosocial needs of refugee children and youth and best practices for filling these needs: a systematic review. Clin Child Psychol Psychiatr 2017;23(2):186–208.
5. Lustig SL, Kia-Keating M, Knight WG, et al. Review of child and adolescent refugee mental health. J Am Acad Child Adolesc Psychiatr 2004;43(1):24–36.
6. American academy of child and adolescent psychiatry (AACAP) committee on community-based systems of care and AACAP committee on quality issues. Electronic address: clinical@aacap.org, American academy of child and adolescent psychiatry (AACAP) committee on community-based systems of care and AACAP committee on quality issues. Clinical update: child and adolescent behavioral health care in community systems of care. J Am Acad Child Adolesc Psychiatr 2022;S0890-8567(22):00291X.
7. Pumariega AJ, Rogers K, Rothe E. Culturally competent systems of care for children's mental health: advances and challenges. Community Ment Health J 2005; 41(5):539–55.
8. Henry-Noel N, Bishop M, Gwede CK, et al. Mentorship in medicine and other health professions. J Cancer Educ 2019;34(4):629–37.
9. Rapp CA, Goscha RJ. The strengths model: case management with people with psychiatric disabilities. 2nd Edition. Oxford: Oxford University Press; 2006.
10. Sierau S, Schneider E, Nesterko Y, et al. Alone, but protected? Effects of social support on mental health of unaccompanied refugee minors. Eur Child Adolesc Psychiatr 2018;28(6):769–80.
11. Soltan F, Uphoff E, Newson R, et al. Community-based interventions for improving mental health in refugee children and adolescents in high-income countries.

Cochrane Database Syst Rev 2020. https://doi.org/10.1002/14651858.cd013657. Published online June 25.

12. Sams DP, Garrison D, Bartlett J. Innovative strength-based care in child and adolescent inpatient psychiatry. J Child Adolesc Psychiatr Nurs 2016;29(3): 110–7.

13. Durlak JA, Wells AM. Primary prevention mental health programs for children and adolescents: a meta-analytic review. Am J Community Psychol 1997;25(2): 115–52.

14. DiClemente K, Sarah Elizabeth N, Berent JM, et al. Understanding mechanisms of change in a family-based preventive mental health intervention for refugees by refugees in New England. Transcult Psychiatr 2022;60(1):142–55.

15. Weine SM. Developing preventive mental health interventions for refugee families in resettlement. Fam Process 2011;50(3):410–30.

16. Im H, Rodriguez C, Grumbine JM. A multitier model of refugee mental health and psychosocial support in resettlement: toward trauma-informed and culture-informed systems of care. Psychol Serv 2020;18(3). https://doi.org/10.1037/ser0000412.

17. Park M, Chesla C, Kit). Understanding complexity of Asian American family care practices. Arch Psychiatr Nurs 2010;24(3):189–201.

Moving?

Make sure your subscription moves with you!

To notify us of your new address, find your **Clinics Account Number** (located on your mailing label above your name), and contact customer service at:

Email: journalscustomerservice-usa@elsevier.com

800-654-2452 (subscribers in the U.S. & Canada)
314-447-8871 (subscribers outside of the U.S. & Canada)

Fax number: 314-447-8029

Elsevier Health Sciences Division
Subscription Customer Service
3251 Riverport Lane
Maryland Heights, MO 63043

*To ensure uninterrupted delivery of your subscription, please notify us at least 4 weeks in advance of move.

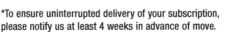
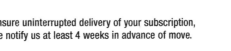

ELSEVIER

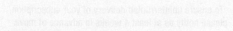

Printed and bound by CPI Group (UK) Ltd, Croydon, CR0 4YY
03/10/2024
01040477-0017